Get Well Soon

The 8 Habits of Healthy People

To: _____

From: _____

Get Well Soon

The 8 Habits of Healthy People

Matt McConnell

Published by True Health Corporation

First printing 2009

ISBN: 978-0-578-01238-4

For my best friend.
Every hour I stole for this book, I stole from you.
Thank you.

Resources supporting this book are available on:

www.habitsofhealth.com

Table of Contents

Introduction

While driving her to school one autumn day, my daughter asked me, "Why did Granddad have to get cancer?" I could tell that she had considered this and worked it around in her head since we had explained that Granddad was sick with something called *cancer*. The human brain is marvelous in its learning instinct. As if lonely from desolation, our young brains automatically seek order and knowledge to fill their wide open, boundless spaces. This seeking instinct shows up as insatiable curiosity in kids and they are prone to asking questions that we, as adults, no longer dare to ask. She just could not make sense of why he *had to have* something that made him sick enough to see the doctor every week.

As adults, we have been given answers – right or wrong – that satisfy our curiosity. As an adult, my brain had been given the knowledge that cancer, and disease in general, is mostly the result of bad luck and poor genetics. Since surviving cancer myself, I had developed a nagging suspicion about the disease and kept a curious eye on it – the statistics, the drugs, the media stories, the finances – but couldn't quite put the pieces together in my mind. Mostly, I was haunted by the great irony of ever-declining health in an ever-modernizing society. It seemed counter-intuitive.

Like a light that turns on in an unfamiliar, empty room to reveal the furniture that had been mere shapes in the dark, her question shined on the formless shapes in a room in my mind.
This time, a bit louder, she asked again, "Daddy, why did Granddad have to get cancer?"

To her, the answer probably seemed routine. But for me, it defined the purpose for my life from that moment on. "He didn't," I said. "He didn't."

Cancer has profoundly affected my life. I suffered from cancer and now suffer from the after effects of its treatment. Cancer ravaged the two men that meant the most to me in my life – my maternal grandfather and my father. Two aunts, three uncles and two grandmothers also suffered from the awful disease and the effects of the treatments used to extend their lives. I am deeply saddened by the suffering and deaths of the millions of innocent people stricken by cancer and other chronic illnesses.

Since being cured of cancer in 1989, I have observed the pervasive sickness that surrounds me with increasing suspicion. The list of serious illnesses that seems, for many, unavoidable – heart disease, stroke, cancer, high blood pressure, Alzheimer's, osteoporosis, dementia – is far too long and far too common, in my opinion, to occur naturally. My daughter's wonderful curiosity was the catalyst that helped me break the barriers that I had built in my own mind and accept that Granddad did not *have* to get cancer.

Contrary to everything we are accustomed to believing, the advancement of civilization has not been all positive, particularly in the area of human health. Sure, because of modern medicine, we are less likely to die of the black plague or the influenza virus, but because of modern eating, drinking and activity habits, we are more likely to get degenerative diseases than we were in the past. Because of mass agriculture, taste bud marketing, convenience food and our fast-paced lives, the health of our species has deteriorated as we have modernized.

Ever since the day I was diagnosed with cancer nearly twenty years ago, I have done extensive research into sickness, health, conventional medicine, alternative medicine and nutrition. I have read countless books, articles and studies, attended seminars, watched videos and listened to audio from medical doctors, alternative healers, cancer survivors, Christian faith authors and health-focused laypeople. As a result of this study, I have become convinced that health is a choice. More specifically, I have become convinced that the poor choices we make accumulate in our bodies and affect everything from hair loss to headaches to hypertension to heart disease.

Human health, it turns out, is the result of human habits. And, unfortunately, the habits that most men, women and children now follow in the civilized world create the perfect storm for the degeneration of the human body, leading to sickness and ultimately to disease. This is bad news, indeed. However, it is far better news than what we have heard from the medical community about most chronic disease, which is, "We're not sure what causes it." If our health is a result of our habits, we can control our health and prevent the sickness and disease that has reached epidemic proportions and ravaged so many of our loved ones.

The eight habits in the pages that follow are, in my opinion, a cure for whatever ails you, but unlike the infomercials that you see on TV, there are no gimmicks. We would all rather take a pill and receive perfect health, but let me be clear: that will not happen. There are no shortcuts to health. Health is a process, not an event. It is a state that is constantly being improved or broken down by the lifestyle choices that you make 20-30 times every day.

This book will help you adopt the eight habits that can restore your body to its natural state. Adopting these habits will put you in control of your health instead of becoming a victim of it. In this book, you will find the habits that have made people healthy for centuries. The same habits recommended for preventing cancer help you control your weight. The same habits that reduce blood pressure help prevent heart disease. The same habits that help prevent Alzheimer's and dementia reduce the risk of arthritis and adult-onset diabetes. These are the habits the body was meant to follow and the rulebook for operating the human machine.

Isn't that what we all want? Which of you reading these words does not fear an abrupt ending to your life from a heart attack, stroke or cancer? Which of you does not worry about aging with sore, swollen joints, high blood pressure and a mind that is slipping away?

These habits can genuinely transform your health and I am living proof. I believe that the contents of this book can have a significant impact on the lives of many, many people who are sick or who will become sick. My hope is that this book can make a difference in the quality of your life and that you will use the knowledge that you gain here to influence the quality of the lives of the people around you.

Get Well Soon!
Matt

P.S. – Please make use of the many free tools and resources that support this book on the Get Well Soon website (www.habitsofhealth.com).

PART I

The Truth about Health

Chapter 1

The Epidemic Secret

Those who think they have no time for healthy living will sooner or later have to find time for illness.

Edward Stanley

"He's not going to make it," the doctor said as he scanned the roomful of faces for a reaction. Everyone froze. He shook his head from side to side, "He's not going to make it."

It was like a dream. Time stopped. Everyone stood motionless and tried to process the news. I lay in the hospital bed, stoned on pain medicine but alert enough to realize that Dr. Headlines had skipped the class on bedside manner.

The thump of my mother's limp body hitting the tile floor broke the silence. She fainted or passed out - I'm not sure I know the difference - but everyone began tending to her. The nurses, my family and even Dr. Headlines scurried about to make sure that she was comfortable. It was a convenient distraction for everyone, actually. No one could muster the courage to look at me.

I remember being unable to think. They say that your life flashes before your eyes when you learn that you are going to die, but I couldn't get my brain to process anything into thoughts or conclusions. I just sat there listening to noises and watching what was going on around me like it was a movie. If my life flashed before my eyes in that moment, it seemed as if there hadn't been very much to it.

I knew that cancer was a terrible diagnosis, but I didn't realize that cancer is not simply one disease. It's hundreds of diseases, making it extremely complex to understand and treat. The American Cancer Society defines cancer as, "a group of diseases characterized by uncontrolled growth and spread of abnormal cells. If the spread is not controlled, it can result in death."

A cancer is actually created when your body reproduces cells, which happens about 70 million times per day, and makes an error, which creates a mutated cell. Cancer is caused by abnormalities in a cell's DNA (its genetic "blueprint"). These may be inherited from parents (5% - 10% of cancers), or they may be caused by outside exposures to carcinogens such as chemicals, radiation, or even infectious organisms (90% - 95% of cancers). The majority of the errors in cell reproduction are actually caught by your immune system. So, in theory, the stronger your immune system, the better your chances are at never developing cancer.

My immune system had a very French approach to defending me. It seemed to simply step aside whenever an invading organism wanted to occupy my body. Ever since I could remember, I caught whatever was going around. I was always missing school and became sick with some form of the flu five to seven times per year.

My flu typically came on fast, showing up first as drowsiness and lightheadedness. Within 24 hours, I would develop a sore throat and congestion. Within 48 hours, I would have difficulty swallowing and enough congestion to create an earache. After about four days or so creating havoc in my head, my cold would then head south to my chest. Once there, I would develop a severe cough and shortness of breath. All of this, of course, was accompanied by a generally lousy state – aches and pains, drowsiness, loss of appetite, etc.

My illnesses would loiter too. Once a cold reached my chest, it seemed to hang out there for weeks. It would not necessarily be severe, but I would have fluid in my lungs for what seemed like an eternity. I even developed a tick of sorts. I was always clearing my throat and lungs because of this fluid, "uhh humm… uhhhh hhhuuummmmmm… uhmm." I guess it became my trademark because my friends would kid me about it. In school, my teachers would glare at me during tests, thinking that I was doing it on purpose and my friends stopped inviting me to play golf with them because I would unconsciously clear my throat during their backswings.

At about age fifteen, I discovered self-medicating. We always had antibiotics around the house and I became an ardent believer in their effectiveness. If I caught it early enough, I could usually knock out a cold with just a few days' doses of antibiotics. By the age of eighteen, I had learned to keep them with me at all times. I always had a stash of something-*acilin* in the glove box of my car. I had to keep them around because I could not afford to miss class (or parties, or dates, or football games). But I continued to get sick so often that I literally became dependent on antibiotics. They became my crutch.

I wasn't unsanitary and I wasn't exposed to more illnesses than the average person. I didn't work in the salt mines and I got plenty of sleep. I lived in a decent neighborhood, attended your average public schools, had yearly physicals and didn't eat lead paint chips. I got plenty of exercise, didn't smoke and I didn't live near power lines or a stream fed by nuclear reactor runoff. I ate what my Mom brought home from the grocery store and I didn't have any more stress than the next guy. So why was I such a sickly person and how did I get cancer?

After being diagnosed, I was asked a lot about my family's history with cancer. At that point, none of my close relatives had ever had cancer. I was the first. Following my diagnosis however, many close relatives have developed different forms of the disease. Cancer literally went up my family tree, starting from the young (me) and moving to the old (my blood-related grandfather, grandmothers, father, uncles and aunts). It turns out that my family is, as the doctors say, genetically predisposed.

Other than us though, the rest of my genetically predisposed family have not become sick. So, what have we done differently than the dozens of other family members who have not gotten sick? Was it simply bad luck or had we pulled some chemical or biological trigger to start the formation of cancer in our bodies that the others had not?

On the surface, I was a typical American boy. I was a relatively active kid, enjoyed playing sports and I was never overweight. I ate the standard American diet - breakfast cereals, lunch meat, hamburgers, tuna fish, pizza, French fries, pancakes, crackers, candy, soda, pastries, etc. Like many teenagers today, I experimented with alcohol and tobacco. None of this was highly unusual or out of the ordinary, however. I was like most every other kid I knew.

So why was I so sick all of the time and how did I wind up with cancer? I used to tease my mother that I was so often sick because she didn't breast feed me. Although most scientists agree that breastfeeding improves a baby's immune function, I am certain that my lack of breast milk was not the cause of my frequent illness or my cancer. Something else was going on.

What I realize now, after nearly twenty years of studying health in order to improve my own, is that being a typical American boy with a typical American lifestyle *was* the problem. My habits, absolutely normal by today's standards, had suppressed my immune system and weakened my defenses. I had become a walking head cold and I substituted antibiotics for my weakened immune system. My lifestyle had damaged my (allegedly genetically predisposed) cells' DNA and millions of mutated cells were being created in my body. A healthy immune system would have identified the mutated cells and attacked them, eliminating them before they could become a tumor, but my immune system was simply not up to the job.

Not long after I started my first year of college, a lump about the size of the tip of a thumb formed on my testicle. It wasn't uncomfortable, but I knew immediately something was wrong. I told my mother and she rushed me to see the urologist near our home in Atlanta. Following a short examination, this doctor explained that my lump was a minor medical problem and nothing to get too concerned about. He suggested that I take warm baths. Warm baths!

After thirty days under his expert guidance, my lump had doubled in size and had become quite uncomfortable. I had lost my appetite and was losing weight. I could barely manage to sit down because of the discomfort, preferring instead to stand and lean against a wall.

Alarmed at my worsening condition, my mother identified the state's top urologist and got me in to see him at his next available appointment – ironically, Friday, January 13th, 1989. This doctor immediately identified my problem as either a tumor or a cist and insisted that we do surgery to remove my testicle that night. A heavy load for an eighteen-year old, I asked if I could have the weekend to be with my friends.

Bright and early Monday morning, I turned up at the hospital to "have my nut cut out," as my warm and sensitive college mates would later say. The surgery went fine, apparently, and I awoke in the recovery room a few hours later. I vividly remember my first thought as I opened my eyes and saw my brother staring down at me: *pain.* Pure, white, searing, freshly-cut pain. When the staff had me sign all of the documents that eliminated them from liability should they cut out the wrong organ, they conveniently failed to tell me that I would not receive any pain medicine until after I woke up as the narcotics could interfere with my sedation.

I did eventually get some pain medicine and the day or so following my surgery is kind of a fog. They wheeled me around in my bed from test to test – CT scan, blood work, MRI, chest x-ray, etc. My extended family had congregated in my hospital room when Dr. Headlines turned up again to deliver the cheerful news – the biopsy of my lump revealed that it was a malignant tumor and the CT scans and MRI showed cancer activity in my abdomen. A urologist, Dr. Headlines had no business prognosticating about my chances with this cancer, but it was just the excitement he was looking for in the otherwise mundane routine of bladder infections and genital warts. I laugh every time I think about him standing in the doorway of my hospital room announcing my imminent death and looking around at the faces of my family like he was waiting for a reaction to the punch line of a poorly rehearsed joke. He came expecting emotion and he got it.

While under the misdiagnosis of my first doctor, the cancer had spread from my testicle into the lymph nodes in my abdomen. I had what my oncologist called stage II testicular cancer. I would need at least three rounds of chemotherapy and would lose my hair and a year of my life fighting the disease. But I would live.

Obviously, I survived the cancer (and the toxins the doctors used to fight the cancer). I temporarily lost my hair, my eyebrows, my sense of taste and about 25 pounds. But I did survive and I became a new person. My cancer gave birth to an activist suspicion about health that would change my life forever.

Losing the War
Motivated by a conviction that I would eventually die from one degenerative disease or another, and a nagging suspicion about the decline of human health in general, I embarked on a study of health that has lasted now for nearly twenty years. Naturally, I began my study by learning everything I could about cancer.

It doesn't take long to discover that more than 1.3 million Americans are diagnosed with cancer every year. However, this raw number lacks context, making it far less shocking than it should be. Annually, it is the equivalent of the entire population of Idaho or New Hampshire or Hawaii getting sick. Imagine that. Stop for a few seconds and imagine if every resident of Idaho developed cancer next year followed by every resident of New Hampshire two years from now and then every resident of Hawaii in three years. Would that seem like a large number of people? Do you think that cancer would have our undivided attention? Mathematically, this is what is happening. It's just not localized to a particular state.

And as we all know, cancer is not simply a medical inconvenience. I discovered that cancer accounts for one out of every 12 deaths in developed countries, and in the U.S., it is now the top killer of Americans under 85 years old. Over 570,000 people died from the disease in 2005.

This number, too, lacks the appropriate context to get our serious attention. Think about this: every minute, an American dies from cancer. At least ten people have died from cancer since you started reading this book. Every month, an entire football stadium full of Americans dies from cancer. Imagine that.

I have often heard that we are "winning the war on cancer," but given the frequency of the disease in the people around me, I was always suspicious of the statement. For a while, I convinced myself that I was just more aware of cancer because I had had it. Over time though, cancer has seemed too prevalent and too persistent a topic with those around me for this to possibly be true.

If someone told you today that we were winning the war on *drugs*, would you be inclined to believe them based on the evidence around you? I certainly see more drug problems among people I know and their families than I have ever seen in my lifetime.

It turns out that my feelings about cancer were right. Cancer is *kicking our butts*. Humankind is losing the war on cancer, but that is not what you read and hear in the press.

There are those who would rather that the public not know this because it puts them at professional risk. I know that sounds like a conspiracy, but let me try to prove this one: both the National Cancer Institute and the American Cancer Society regularly produce a chart entitled "Cancer Death Rates." In this chart, they plot the death rate per 100,000 people for the leading types/ sites of cancer (lung & bronchus, prostate, colon & rectum, breast, etc.) over some period going back to at least the 1970's.

Viewing cancer this way shows a tremendous reduction in deaths per 100,000 for the leading types of cancer since the mid 1980's.

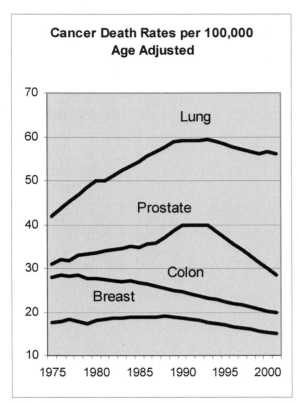

Cancer Death Rates per 100,000
Age Adjusted

Viewing the chart, placed so prevalently throughout the NCI and ACS literature (order the latest Cancer Facts & Figures booklet from the American Cancer Society and it is always on page 2 or 3) leads the reader to believe that, since death from cancer is down, cancer must be down. However, if you research cancer *incidence* (the number of people that actually get the disease), it has increased significantly over the time periods covered by the Cancer Death Rate charts.

In the early 1900's, the average American had a 1 in 50 chance of getting cancer. Today, 1 in 3 can expect to get cancer in their lifetime; 1 in every 2 males. One in eight women living today will develop breast cancer. Not too long ago, it was one in ten. Can you imagine what that chart would look like? Are you surprised that neither this chart nor the data show up prominently in the NCI or ACS literature?

From 1990 through 2006 there were over 22 million new cases of cancer in the United States. That equates to roughly 7% of the entire U.S. population in just 16 years. Incredibly, the statisticians at USA Today estimate that by 2015, seven short years from the publishing of this book, 78% of Americans will have had cancer, or will some day be facing it.

So, if cancer incidence is way up, but death rates are decreasing, what does this mean? How can incidence go up and death rates go down simultaneously? It is a result of advances in cancer *treatments* to deal with the disease once it occurs.

In other words, when cancer occurs today, fewer people die from it than two decades ago because we have improved the treatment of cancer symptoms, namely tumors. So, people are getting the disease in ever-greater numbers, but we can now treat them once they do. Is that "winning the war on cancer?" How could anyone make the claim that we are "winning a war" when 1) the "enemy" is attacking and harming more victims than ever before, and 2) the "enemy" is still killing one person every minute? I think the only people winning in this war are in the treatment business.

This tactic isn't exclusive to cancer. In January of 2008, CNN Evening News celebrated a report that deaths from heart disease and stroke were down more than 25%, well ahead of the 2010 goals set by the American Heart Association. The newscast went on to say that this great victory was due to advances in medical technology like stints and angioplasty and medications for treating high cholesterol, high blood pressure and blood clots. I sat and wondered if other people had heard what I had. The newscasters really seemed to buy the propaganda they were parroting, but I wondered if John Q Public was convinced. Isn't this a lot like the business news declaring that the economy is healthy by pointing out that there are fewer business bankruptcies as a result of government bail-outs?

Imagine if President George W. Bush had announced that America was "winning the war" in Iraq and showed a chart to the American public plotting the decreasing death rates for different types of war wounds (gunshot, explosions, shrapnel, etc.). Now, imagine if you found out that significantly more Americans were actually being shot, blown up and wounded by shrapnel than ever before in the Iraq war, but advances in field medicine were able to keep them alive longer. They were being wounded and maimed by the enemy in ever-increasing numbers, but advances in medicine were now able to keep them alive. Would you feel like we were winning that war? Would you be angry that our president, the Commander in Chief of the war effort, measured success based on improvements in the medical treatment of our ever-increasing wounded?

And if you think that comparing cancer patients to soldiers maimed by terrorists is unfair, you need only visit the cancer floor at your local hospital or volunteer at an oncology camp for kids to see the stunning similarities. Cancer and the terrorists' Improvised Explosive Devices (IEDs) create the same wounds. Like an IED, surgery and radiation to repair brain tumors can leave patients without hearing and eyesight, stunt mental development and growth, and can severely disfigure the victim. Like an IED, bone cancer can cost victims their arms and/or legs. Like an IED, cancer in the organs or the blood can cause victims to lose bodily functions and spend the rest of their lives connected to tubes, bags, machines and prescriptions. Unlike an IED, however, when a victim is killed by cancer, he is killed slowly and, often, painfully. These aren't patients – they are victims. Just like soldiers attacked by terrorists.

All of this makes me think unpopular thoughts about the National Cancer Institute and the American Cancer Society (like maybe they should change their names to the National Cancer *Treatment* Institute and the American Cancer *Treatment* Society). It makes me wonder what they are really spending their time and *our* money doing. If they are able to justify their continued existence (and salaries) as a result of advances in treatment after the "enemy" attacks, how much time, money and effort do they put into preventing the "enemy" from attacking? More specifically, if public concern can be placated by a graph and well-placed news stories that report a decrease in death rates over the last couple of decades – and they continue to receive funding and their paychecks as a result – why should they emphasize prevention, an area where the forty-year graphs look awful? It also makes me wonder who the biggest beneficiaries of these organizations are if they justify their existence and derive their success largely from advances in cancer treatments. I am afraid I know the answer, but voicing it is about as trendy as burning the flag.

The bottom line is that we are *not* currently winning the war on drugs, we are *not* winning the war in Iraq, and we are *not* winning the war on cancer. For that matter, as you will see, we are not winning the war on heart disease, arthritis, dementia, diabetes, hypertension or any degenerative disease. We are losing them all.

Cancer is all around us and it is obvious, without even knowing the statistics above, that its incidence is increasing rapidly. In 1971, when I was one-year old, President Richard Nixon declared war on cancer and we've never been whipped so decisively. In my lifetime, cancer has grown exponentially. It is rampant and the best defenses we have are cutting, burning and poisoning ourselves. If the trend continues unchecked, I suppose we can expect cancer to be as common as poor eyesight, but far less treatable.

The Disease Epidemic

If you were to randomly select 100 Americans and study them, statistics suggest that you would find a very unhealthy group:

- 5 have diagnosed diabetes and another 5 have diabetes and don't know it
- 24 have high blood pressure
- 27 have cardiovascular disease
- 33 have had or will have cancer
- 33 are obese
- 70 are overweight

If you extrapolate those numbers across the population of the United States, then you find that 72 million Americans have high blood pressure, 81 million have cardiovascular disease and 99 million have or will have cancer. The numbers are staggering in a country with a total population of only 300 million.

It should not be a surprise to learn, then, that the top three causes of death in the United States are heart disease (killing over 650,000 per year), cancer (killing nearly 600,000 per year) and stroke (killing over 150,000 per year). Americans have a higher likelihood of dying from these diseases than people who live in other parts of the world, too. For example, with less than 1/20th of the world's population, America has 1/12th of the world's heart disease deaths. I'm no statistician, but I think that means that if you live in America, you have a much greater chance of dying from heart disease than the population of the rest of the world – and it could easily be argued that the U.S. has the world's best health care system. Think about that for a second. The world's highest per capita incidence of heart disease is concentrated in the world's only superpower: the United States of America.

While the big three affect an enormous number of people in the United States, other chronic illnesses and health conditions are growing at an unprecedented rate here as well. Rounding out the top seven causes of death in the United States (after heart disease, cancer and stroke) are chronic lower respiratory disease, accidents, diabetes and Alzheimer's disease. Today, approximately 16 million people have Type II diabetes and the number is expected to double by 2025. Some 4.5 million Americans have Alzheimer's disease and the number is expected to reach 13 million by 2050. Another 49 million people have been diagnosed with arthritis, making it the leading cause of disability in the United States. Incredibly, one out of every 200 people in the United States gets Parkinson's disease and the number of cases of Autism has doubled in the last ten years so that, today, 1 in 160 kids born are diagnosed with autism. Even allergies - dairy, peanut, pollen, dust, etc - have become as common as tooth decay. More than 50 million Americans suffer from allergies.

I am deeply concerned about the scale of the sickness epidemic in our country. In our modern era, with all of our resources, it seems ludicrous to think that we are actually getting *sicker* as a species. We can transplant human organs, adjust eyesight with lasers and surgically limit the effects of aging. We can build a functioning mechanical heart, re-grow hair and help the profoundly deaf to hear. But we can't put a dent in the epidemic of degenerative disease. It seems that health itself is becoming extinct.

In the media, I continually hear references to people living longer, healthier lives thanks to modern medicine. We are lulled into believing that we are healthier because the average life expectancy continues to increase. We are either unduly proud of our ability to treat sickness and disease after it occurs or we are victims of the aggressive marketing of special interests. Either way, I don't buy that we are healthier.

Look around! Average life expectancy might be up, but, like the cancer example above, so is incidence. We are sick. Chronic illness and degenerative disease have reached epidemic proportions.

In the years since my illness, one of my grandmothers and an aunt were diagnosed with breast cancer, an uncle had prostate cancer, and my grandfather and my Dad died of liver cancer. Another grandfather died of heart disease. On my wife's side, one grandmother died from Alzheimer's and another died of liver cancer. I have uncles who have had strokes and others are dealing with high blood pressure, heart disease, high cholesterol and Chron's disease. And it's not just me. My friends have similar stories. In the last year alone, one friend's 33-year old brother and another friend's 50-something-year old wife were diagnosed with ALS (Lou Gehrig's disease). Another friend's husband was diagnosed with Parkinson's disease and three others have spouses who are fighting cancer.

Sometimes, I feel like we're part of this great marketing conspiracy. I really do. I know I sound like some weirdo sitting in the desert in Roswell, New Mexico, waiting for the government to slip up and reveal the alien space station that's been hidden in hangar 11 since before the first man (allegedly) walked on the moon. But it just doesn't compute for me why the media is reporting that we are living longer and healthier when it seems like they should be ringing the alarm bells and screaming about the epidemic of degenerative disease in the developed world. Strangely, I feel a little bit like a citizen in a country where the media is controlled by the state (or business) and I am being told the news according to the political (or financial) interests controlling the media. Maybe I am naïve and idealistic, but I feel that the media has a responsibility to report this stuff, not just reprint Pfizer's press releases.

Even if the media was widely reporting the truth about health, it would take time to convince the public. As beings created in the image of our God, we want to believe that we are making progress. We want to believe that we are healthier. We don't want to think that we are going backwards in any area, particularly not the health of our species. We want to believe in human ingenuity and man's dominion over the earth and everything in it. It took a long time for people to begin to admit that we were destroying the earth's environment and its atmosphere, but we eventually did because of overwhelming scientific evidence. The same data exists about the epidemic of disease overtaking our species. We simply need to review the evidence and the truth will emerge from the propaganda.

In 2007, I launched an online survey called The Preventive Health Survey. The response was terrific and the data enlightening. As a result, I will be expanding the survey and conducting it annually. I have included the 2007 survey data in different sections throughout this book and the survey data regarding the incidence of sickness are below. When asked which chronic illnesses had afflicted their friends and relatives most often, survey respondents chose cancer, heart disease and high blood pressure, in that order.

How many of your relatives and friends have been afflicted with the following chronic illnesses?

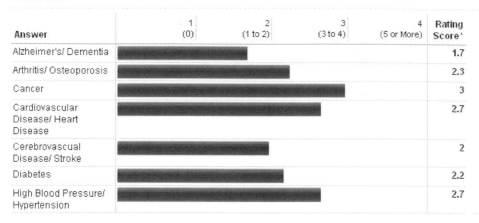

Answer	1 (0)	2 (1 to 2)	3 (3 to 4)	4 (5 or More)	Rating Score
Alzheimer's/ Dementia					1.7
Arthritis/ Osteoporosis					2.3
Cancer					3
Cardiovascular Disease/ Heart Disease					2.7
Cerebrovascular Disease/ Stroke					2
Diabetes					2.2
High Blood Pressure/ Hypertension					2.7

Not surprisingly, when asked in a separate question which conditions respondents were most concerned about affecting their own health, the majority answered that they were most concerned about cancer and heart disease. Interestingly though, most also reported that they are as concerned about arthritis and Alzheimer's as they are about high blood pressure, even though their friends and relatives aren't as afflicted with arthritis and Alzheimer's. This seems to indicate either a sincere concern regarding one's old age lifestyle or a genuine fear of these two conditions from firsthand experience with friends or relatives.

When asked how many of their close friends and relatives had passed away as a result of chronic illness, 64% of survey respondents said that they had lost three or more friends and relatives to chronic illness and 30% reported losing five or more.

In total, how many of your relatives and friends have passed away as a result of chronic illnesses listed in the question above?

Answer	0%	100%	Response Ratio
0			5%
1 to 2			28%
3 to 4			34%
5 to 6			15%
7 or More			15%

Where is the public outrage? Why haven't ratings-starved news outlets broken stories and fund-starved universities commissioned studies and vote-starved politicians campaigned on this issue? More importantly, what is causing this epidemic and how can it be stopped?

Chapter 2

How Science and Profit Abducted Health

Health is a state of complete physical, mental and social well-being, and not merely the absence of disease or infirmity.

World Health Organization, 1948

In sports, preventative medicine is used to prevent sports injuries. In professional football, for example, ankles, wrists, fingers and knees are taped, neck braces and padded helmets are worn, and cut blocking and helmet-to-helmet contact are not allowed. This is done because the rule-makers in the National Football League can directly link causes – like helmet-to-helmet contact – to outcomes – like concussions. As a result, the league and the teams are able to take steps to prevent the causes of injuries and protect their players.

In human health, by contrast, there are plenty of outcomes. But unlike professional football, there are far fewer direct links to causes. When someone turns up in a doctor's office with recurring migraine headaches, for example, it is not as easy as running an instant replay to find the cause. The human body is incredibly complex and the environment in which each one operates can be dramatically different. To get a better understanding of what is going on with the patient, doctors will take the patient's vital signs, ask questions, conduct a short examination, and may even run some blood work or order an X-ray, MRI or CT scan. However, these are relatively blunt instruments in the search for causes to problems in the highly complex human organism. The origin of migraine headaches and so many other human ailments exceed the sophistication of the tools that doctors have to diagnose them.

As advanced as we think we are, our science is simply not mature enough to isolate causes in a setting with so many variables. When you hear western doctors and scientists say, "We do not know what causes [this or that condition]," it is an acknowledgement that the complexity of the human body exceeds the sophistication of current science. Modern western medicine is able to manage trauma, treat medical emergencies, treat bacterial infections, prevent many infectious diseases with immunization, replace worn out or damaged body parts (hips, knees, hearts, etc.), and get good results with cosmetic surgery. However, modern western medicine is *not* capable of curing most chronic degenerative disease, autoimmune disease, neurological disease, mental illness, allergy or viral infection.

I would argue that there is enough empirical evidence about the causes of many of these conditions and an overwhelming need to act in the interest of the public to take a few leaps over the gaps that modern science leaves (this is where the scientists will cringe). But modern medicine chooses instead to emphasize the alleviation of the symptoms that result from these conditions. Science has become, after all, the backbone of medicine and deviation from it, however immature our science may be in comparison to the human body, seems to be out of the question.

Symptoms, like the dilation of blood vessels in the brain during a migraine, are more easily diagnosed and treated than the environmental triggers that *cause* the blood vessels in the brain to dilate, for example. Because diagnosing and treating the *symptoms* (the outcomes) of a condition are within the sophistication of modern science and the identification of the *causes* of the condition are not, western medicine emphasizes the treatment of symptoms over the elimination of causes. While this type of medicine alleviates discomfort in patients, it does not alleviate the cause of the condition. Symptoms, like a fever or a headache, help us to know that something is wrong. Removing the symptom blinds us to the fact that something is causing a problem in our body.

Interestingly, symptom alleviation is also more easily 'productized' than cause prevention. Developing and selling a pill to constrict blood vessels in the brain is far more scalable and profitable than giving someone a worksheet to help them document the environmental factors that might trigger their headaches. Given the maturity of our science, the medical industry has figured out that it is easier to make money treating the symptoms of sickness than in preventing the causes of it.

As a result, most of us living in the western hemisphere associate medicine with symptom relief. When we visit the doctor, we're happy to get a symptom-reducing prescription to relieve our high blood pressure, cholesterol, inflammation, etc. We don't really think about causes when dealing with our own health. It is as if we have been brainwashed into thinking that causes are out of our control or simply too complex to consider.

Can you imagine taking your smoking car to the mechanic and him giving you a fan to blow the smoke out of the cabin while you drive? Can you imagine calling a plumber about a leak in your basement and him installing a drain in the basement floor? It wouldn't happen. The mechanic would search out and fix the cause of the smoke and the plumber would find and fix the cause of the leak. But that is not what typically happens in western medicine. At the doctor's office, you often get symptom suppression instead of cause identification and elimination. And, worst of all, in nearly every case, patients are okay with it! They accept it without a second thought.

Why Prevention is Better Than Symptom Treatment
It is important to understand the distinctions between the words here. Generally speaking, an illness or condition will have one or more causes and one or more outcomes (or symptoms). *Treatments* typically don't do anything about the causes of a condition. Treatments correct or address the outcomes or symptoms of a condition without eliminating them. A simple example of a treatment is the use of corrective eye glasses for nearsightedness.

Similarly, *cures* typically don't do anything about the causes of an illness or condition. Cures do, however, eliminate one or more outcomes of an illness or condition. A simple example of a cure is refractive laser eye surgery, or Lasik. This surgery can correct the malformations in the eye. Another example would be the chemotherapy drugs that I was given to kill the cancer in my body.

As the name implies, *prevention* is any activity to avoid that which causes an illness or condition (there are other definitions of prevention that the medical community uses once a disease process is active, but for the purposes of this book, I use the word prevention as defined above). Prevention focuses on the causes of an illness or condition. Prevention indirectly addresses outcomes or symptoms by eliminating causes, but prevention does not directly go after outcomes or symptoms. An example of prevention would be eye exercises to prevent nearsightedness that researchers believe is caused by excessive "near-work" like reading, using a computer or watching television. In this example, effective prevention would eliminate the outcome of nearsightedness and avoid the need for glasses (treatment) or LASIK surgery (cure).

Because treatments and cures address only the outcomes or symptoms of underlying causes of sickness and disease, I think they fall drastically short as the primary tools used in modern western medicine. If you disagree with me, go back and read chapter one of this book again and consider the statistics. Sickness and disease in the western world has reached epidemic proportions and medicine is largely dealing with outcomes. We are putting fans in smoking cars and we can't figure out why so many cars are broken down on the side of the road.

I will admit that cancer drugs eliminated my cancer. I owe my life to the drugs Cisplatin, Vinblastine and Bleomycin. I suffer from the side effects of these poisons, but that is a fair trade for life, in my opinion. The real problem is that I did not change the habits and the lifestyle choices that *caused* my cancer in the first place. After recovering from cancer, I got right back on the path to self-destruction, adding to the cumulative effect that caused my cancer in the first place. Now that we had confirmed that I was predisposed to cancer, someone needed to sit me down and talk to me about cause and effect. I was destined to get sick again.

It seems to me that medical professionals should become more like policemen than firefighters. Medicine should emphasize "crime" prevention, detective work and cause elimination over emergency response, "fire" suppression and damage control. Because treatment merely addresses symptoms and our science isn't nearly sophisticated enough to develop cures for the wide range of complex human disease processes, I believe that we would be better off if the medical profession emphasized cause prevention. In his book *Walking in Divine Health*, Dr. Don Colbert, a practicing medical doctor, says, "Our system is geared to treat medical problems with everything from surgery and medical procedures to cholesterol-lowering drugs and medications... The key to having a healthy future lies not in better medication or more skilled surgeons, but in total prevention."

I am confident that, in time, this will happen. Some day, medical professionals will not simply look at the physical symptoms of a patient and prescribe symptom-suppressing drugs, therapy or surgery. Instead, they will look for the underlying causes for those symptoms and use a variety of approaches to address the causal imbalances in order to return the patient to health. As an example, when reviewing a patient that complains of a skin rash, sore joints and weight loss, instead of prescribing anti-inflammatory or arthritis drugs, health professionals would ideally review all three conditions in search of a common underlying cause, such as a food allergy. Then, only when the cause is determined, health professionals would work to neutralize the cause using the appropriate combination of nutrition, lifestyle changes, conventional and alternative medicine.

Until that happens however, consumers of western medicine have to rethink their health and the role that western medicine plays in it. Many, many people live unhealthy lives with the expectation that medicine will "fix" them when they break down. The reality is that traditional medicine is not equipped to continually fix what it takes years of bad habits to break. Health is complex to destroy and it is complex to fix – more complex than our science can comprehend in most cases.

An Unhealthy Commitment to Science
One of the most prominent astrophysicists of the early 20ᵗʰ century was Sir Arthur Eddington. He made several significant contributions to the area of physics and was one of the first physicists who understood the early ideas of relativity along with Albert Einstein. In fact, Eddington introduced Einstein's theory of relativity to the English-speaking world. Like many of the great minds in early science, Sir Eddington helped to expand science by questioning its limits.

Once, while being critical of the current-day methods of scientific discovery, he is known to have told a parable about a fisherman who used a net with a three-inch mesh. The fisherman spent all of his days fishing in the ocean and observed that all of the fish he caught were longer than three inches. Finally, returning from a day spent fishing with his nets and observing his catch, he proudly declared that he had discovered that there were absolutely no fish in existence shorter than three inches in length.

Eddington's parable was meant to illustrate the limitations of scientific discovery. As you will read in this chapter, the complexity of the human organism far exceeds the sophistication of our scientific measurement. Because of the immaturity of our scientific tools in relation to the human body, I believe that an unwavering commitment to science in the field of human health is a critical flaw that prevents us from discovering truths about human health that are vital to the survival of our species. As in Eddington's parable, I believe that the mesh of our net – what I will generally refer to as "science" – is too wide and that the health equivalent of fish less than three inches are slipping right through it.

However, unlike the fisherman in the parable, medical scientists recognize that their net has large holes and isn't catching everything. Instead of drawing ludicrous conclusions like the fisherman in the parable, most in medicine readily acknowledge that there is a lot in the "ocean" of health that their net isn't able to catch because science has not developed the sophistication required to fully observe and classify the complex human body. For example, how many times have you heard, "We don't know what causes … [Lupus, Chron's disease, Parkinson's disease, migraines, Alzheimer's, attention deficit disorder (ADD), ALS, food allergies, Down's syndrome, epilepsy, Huntington's disease…]"? The mesh in the current net of science is large and, therefore, not helpful in discovering many of the intricate and complicated details about human health – but at least we are willing to admit it.

The problem exists in the fact that the men and women of medicine are largely unwilling to consider using anything else with which to fish for new information about health. There is an unwavering commitment to the net of science and the medical field seems content to wait on it to mature (for the holes in the net of science to get small enough to catch the "smaller" facts about human health). At the current pace of advancement in science, that could take 50, 100, or even 200 years! Given the epidemic of degenerative disease facing our species, that is simply too long to wait. The rate of increase in deadly degenerative disease in humans is far outpacing the rate of scientific advancement. We could be extinct before science matures enough to give us the answers we need!

How Science is Failing Us
It is shocking when you realize how immature we are in medicine today. I think people believe that the medical community's understanding of the human body is much further along than it really is. Cancer treatment is an excellent example. Similar to our current stage in space exploration, we are making great progress and lots of smart people and money are hard at work, but what we *don't* know far exceeds what we *do* know.

Researchers in every field of study, including medicine, rigorously adhere to the principles of science. Science, as defined by Webster's dictionary is, "A branch of study which is concerned with observation and classification of facts, especially with the establishment of verifiable general laws chiefly by induction and hypothesis." Said more simply, science is *a method of making sense of the unknown by observation and classification of facts*.

If, for example, you wanted to understand water, you could use science to observe its freezing and boiling points (32°F and 100°F). You could determine its molecular weight, study its interaction with other substances and so on. Once you have a complete and thorough observation and classification of water's facts, you have a model by which you can make accurate predictions about the behaviors and characteristics of water (you can form laws). If, however, you have an incomplete set of facts about water, you cannot accurately predict its behaviors and characteristics. If all you knew was that water boiled at 100°F, you would not understand how or why ice is formed, for example.

Because the complexity of the human body exceeds the sophistication of our measurement capabilities (more on this below), science has an incomplete set of facts about the human body and, therefore, medicine cannot accurately predict all of the behaviors and characteristics of the human body. That would be fine were it not for two very important points: 1) the medical profession views science as the only legitimate method of discovering the unknown about human health, and 2) science proceeds slowly in complex systems, protracting the discovery of facts and the formation of laws about those systems. In other words, we're committed to riding a tortoise through a forest fire. We know there is a forest fire and we know we're riding a tortoise. There is a small chance that we can escape the forest fire on that tortoise, but we're staying on the tortoise! Shouldn't we be looking for a faster way out?

Too Many Variables
In order to establish a scientific fact, you must create an environment where one variable is studied and all other variables are controlled. Isolating one element of study while controlling all of the other elements in an environment is a requirement to establish scientifically reliable results. And, to be scientifically valid, experiments must provide the same results over and over again.
As a result, science and the scientific method literally stall in complex systems like the economy, the earth's ecosystem and the human body. This is because of the many variables that cannot be isolated while a

single variable is studied for cause and effect. Truth be told, nothing can be scientifically proven about the cause of most disease processes in the human body because our scientific tools are too simple to effectively hold the thousands and thousands of chemical, biological, electrical, emotional and environmental variables constant across the many complex systems of our bodies while individual variables are tested to understand cause and effect. Trying to understand whether Teflon coating from nonstick cookware causes DNA mutation while holding all of the other variables in the body constant (patient history, diet, environment, cell chemistry, organ function, mood, body temperature, sleep patterns, stress, etc.) is impossible today.

Although science is the best means we have to establish absolute facts from the unknown, it is not very helpful until you have a full study of all of the variables of the unknown item that you are observing. Take for example the economy and our ecosystem. Using the science of math (including economics, statistics, probability, etc.), we are unable to create an accurate model of all of the aspects of the U.S. economy because there are far too many variables at play. Using the sciences of physics, biology, chemistry, astronomy, etc., we are unable to create an accurate model of all of the aspects of the earth's ecosystem (we can't even forecast the weather with a great degree of accuracy) because there are far too many variables at play in the ecosystem (and interactions among variables and interactions from interactions). We simply don't have the capacity to isolate and study so many variables. Without the capacity to do this, science simply fails.

That said, a lack of adequate understanding has not stopped an entire industry from prognosticating the movements of the stock market and the broader economy. Neither has it stopped special interest groups from regularly identifying (with great zeal) the exact causes of various ecological woes.

I submit that there are at least as many complex variables at play in the human body as there are in the economy or our ecosystem. The human body is like a puzzle of a million pieces and we have put together, maybe, one hundred thousand pieces. Because there are so many variables, so many puzzle pieces not yet put into place, there is not a set of facts and laws that we can rely upon to consistently make accurate predictions about the behavior and characteristics of the human body and human health.

As a simple example of the successful isolation of variables, consider injuries from auto accidents. The auto industry was able to prove that antilock brakes and airbags save lives. As a result, they are now found on most automobiles. However, there were relatively few variables to control. At a test track, engineers added antilock brakes to cars and the distance that it took those cars to come to a complete stop shortened versus the exact same automobile on the exact same track without antilock brakes. In a crash testing laboratory, engineers added airbags to a certain model car and ran controlled front impact tests and the crash test dummies came out with fewer "injuries" versus the exact same automobiles in the exact same laboratory undergoing the exact same front impact test without front air bags.

Human injuries typically have easily isolated causes and, therefore, it is easy to develop preventive measures to avoid them happening. However, with disease processes inside the human body, it is not as easy to test "additives" like you test antilock brakes or airbags on a car. You cannot simply change a variable like sugar consumption and inspect the outcome. The other variables affecting human health are far too complex and far too many to expect scientifically valid results. Tests of the complex human body are much harder to control than tests of simpler systems. Science requires a controlled environment in which to test and, as control decreases, uncertainty increases. In other words, as a result of a lack of control, it is very difficult to use science to evaluate the affect of individual elements on human health.

Unfortunately for you and me, western civilization associates inexactness with incorrectness. As a result, science is the only discipline that the western medical community will recognize as valid for producing health knowledge, despite the fact that it is unable to uncover the causes of most human sickness today. Said another way, medical scientists trust the tortoise that we are riding through the forest fire because it is sure-footed and unlikely to stumble.

We, the Patients
Medicine's lack of understanding of the human body is not, by itself, a bad thing. In fact, I don't think that the medical community, in general, holds itself out as being more knowledgeable that it is. We, the patients, are the problem.

Most people believe that the medical community has a near complete understanding of the human body. We trust doctors, nurses, hospitals and drug companies with our health because we want to believe that medical professionals know how to cure us and keep us healthy. We fear sickness, injury, death and disease and we want to believe that there is someone who can protect us from it. We want to believe it so badly that our hope has transformed into fact. Although traditional (allopathic) medical doctors spend relatively little time in school learning about preventive health – and despite the fact that there is plenty of preventive health information available from naturopathic health providers and on the Internet – 28% of respondents to the 2007 Preventive Health Survey said they would turn to their traditional medical doctor first when looking for preventive health advice.

As a result of our unquestioning support of the traditional medical industry, we have empowered it to be the single authority on human health. Unfortunately, it isn't. Yes, doctors, nurses, hospitals and drug companies know more about the human body that Joe Public, but they still understand far less than half of what there is to know about the human organism, in my estimation. As an example, relatively little is known about what causes most neurological disorders like Parkinson's disease, Alzheimer's disease, Lou Gehrig's disease, migraines, seizures, depression, etc. Similarly, there is very little scientific confirmation about what causes cancer at a molecular level. The medical industry can treat some of the symptoms from these diseases, but it is absolutely helpless against the causes.

We look at early medical practices like blood-letting and leaches and consider ourselves to be incredibly modern by comparison. In truth, however, using chemicals with dangerous side effects that have no impact on causation, cutting out glands and organs that our creator put into our bodies for a purpose, and consuming animal hormones to slow the inevitable march of time isn't anything to put into a time capsule and brag about. I feel sure that people will look back at our medicine as incredibly primitive in another fifty years.

That said, however, I want to be careful not to vilify the many wonderful people working in the medical industry. Many people enter the medical profession out of love for other human beings. They go into medicine because they want to help heal the sick and injured. These people are genuinely compassionate and deserve our respect for their authentic concern for others. They are people with a calling and a gift to help others and they have sacrificed their lives to serve you and me. Furthermore, I am confident that the people that went into medicine because of their love for their fellow man will willingly entertain a debate about the state and direction of human health.

I simply believe that the medical community needs to step down from the pedestal that we've put them on, lock arms with their fellow man and admit that we have a sickness epidemic that science can't solve fast enough. In its current state of maturity, our science is unable to provide us with the answers that we need. We've tamed the earth and everything on it. We can escape the forest fire, but we've got to get off of the tortoise in order to do it.

Double Standard

The scientific community (and the press that doesn't dare question it) will not, under any circumstances, draw definitive conclusions about the links between human toxicity and chronic disease. When talking about the diseases that plague us today, how many times have you heard, "We are not sure what causes…"? And, when discussing a potentially troubling link between some form of human toxin and a chronic disease, how many times have you read, "There is no scientific evidence to support…"? The scientific community, it seems, will not in any way render an opinion to warn the public about what seems so obvious – that we are not-so-slowly killing ourselves with the lifestyles we've chosen and the toxic surroundings in which we live.

The opposite is not true, however. The scientific community, lacking scientific proof, is very willing to declare that something is *not* killing us. In October, 2006, the media declared "Fish is good!" Two federally funded studies had found that eating one to two servings of fish high in fatty oils per week reduced the risk of heart attack. The studies also assessed the risk of exposure to toxic chemicals in fish such as mercury, dioxins and polychlorinated biphenyls (PCBs) and declared that the health risks for the general public were "inconclusive."

Let me replay that for you: "*Uncontrolled* studies of consumption of fish revealed that fish consumption can prevent heart attacks… Fatty fish oils are good for the heart… So eat up. Fish is good… Oh yea, and the chemical toxins commonly found in fish may not be bad for you because the study was inconclusive…What's that? You want to know why you are sick? We're not sure what causes that… Eat more fish, though… What's that? There are some toxic chemicals in fish and some suspicious links between those toxic chemicals and chronic disease... But, it has not been scientifically proven, right? And our study was *not controlled*, right? Hmmm... Inconclusive... Fish oil is good for the heart... Eat more fish..." These guys either work for the chemical companies or they get paid when you get sick... or both.

Isn't it odd that we need absolutely tangible, repeatable, valid, irrefutable scientific proof that something is killing people before the scientific community is willing to declare it's a danger, but all we need is a preponderance of the evidence to convict a murderer to die in a court of law? Now that is a double standard if I've ever heard of one. In both instances, we are working in a complex system – a human body and a crime scene – to convict a killer, but medicine needs significantly more evidence than the law. In fact, health problems kill far more people than murderers *and* the consequences of a "false conviction" in health are far less severe, so you would think that the burden of proof and the standard of "conviction" in medicine would be the same as it is in law or lower, but not significantly higher.

So, one of the two systems is screwed up. Either medicine needs too much proof or law needs too little. Let's test it by switching the two standards and see what happens:

If, instead of a preponderance of the evidence, you needed absolutely tangible, repeatable, valid, irrefutable scientific proof that someone had committed a murder in order to convict them to die, we would not get many convictions. Murder would be relatively easy to get away with. To be convicted, a person would need to be seen committing the murder by multiple witnesses or get caught on video, leave DNA at the crime scene, and get caught in possession of the weapon.

- *Positives*: Innocent people would not be convicted.

- *Negatives*: Most murderers would never get convicted and they would be free to roam the streets.

- *My Conclusion*: Not a good fit.

If, instead of absolutely tangible, repeatable, valid, irrefutable scientific proof, you needed a preponderance of the evidence that something was a health risk in order to "convict" it, knowledge about human health could progress at a much faster pace. The "case" that has to be made to "convict" a killer with a preponderance of the evidence is far more reasonable than irrefutable scientific evidence.

- *Positives:* Medical science could more quickly "convict" those health risks with strong evidence, safeguarding people from potential harm.

- *Negatives:* We may unnecessarily "convict" certain health risks (foods, ingredients, additives, etc.) and people would avoid them.

- *My Conclusion:* Something to consider. If the alternative is that the standard remains too high and that it takes us a very long time to actually "convict" the real health risks and those health risks are "free to roam the streets" and kill more and more people every year, I vote for a standard of a preponderance of the evidence in medicine, at least until we begin winning the war on degenerative diseases that are ravaging our species.

Clearly, our science cannot move fast enough to catch up with and overtake the sickness epidemic that we have on our hands. It simply isn't mature enough to successfully isolate the cause and effect of the complex disease processes that are occurring in our bodies. This is global warming on a human level and we can't wait 100 years until all of the scientists have the tools to run controlled experiments on humans and nod their heads in unison about the causes of disease. We can't simply watch people suffer and die while we wait around until science matures enough to help us prevent and cure disease. *Unless we make a change* in the way we approach the problem, we are destined to wait and quietly wonder what is killing so many of our friends and relatives.

I believe that we have to shift our burden of proof from indisputable scientific evidence to a preponderance of evidence. Similar to the level of evidence needed to convict killers in a court of law, I think we need to "convict" killers in human health with a preponderance of the evidence. We can do this using the empirical evidence for what is causing disease, basically observed substantiation, instead of requiring controlled, repeatable experiments where all of the untested variables are held constant.

We do have the scientific tools to "convict" causes of human disease using a preponderance of the evidence. We can look at populations of sick people and isolate on the similarities. We can also look at populations of well people and isolate on the habits that keep them well. And what is the worst that could happen? In the course of eliminating those things that *are* likely causing many of the diseases facing mankind, we might falsely "convict" a food additive, a chemical pesticide or an ingredient in the manufacturing of plastics and ban those substances from use. In an effort to prolong the survival of our species, shouldn't some breakage be an acceptable consequence? When you consider that we are dealing with an epidemic, is that really that bad? Is the freedom of enterprise to be protected more than human health?

Take the Leap
Leonardo daVinci is easily one of history's greatest geniuses. He observed and explained more about our complex world with his paintings and drawings than any man before or since. His broad field of study included anatomy, physics, botany, paleontology, astrology, biology, architecture, map making and engineering, to name a few. He was unrivaled in his ability to observe the world around him and discern understanding. He once said, "My works arise from unadulterated and simple experience, which is the one true mistress, the one true muse. The rules of experience are all that is needed to discern the true from the false; experience is what helps all men to look temperately for the possible, rather than cloaking oneself in ignorance."
The "rules of experience" regarding our health are certainly obvious enough that it does not take a man like Leonardo daVinci "to discern the true from the false." The empirical evidence against the lifestyle choices and toxins that are likely killing us is overwhelming. The lifestyles and habits of men and women living in modern countries have deteriorated human health to such an extent that degenerative disease has become an epidemic. For the first time in our history, this generation of children is expected to have a shorter life expectancy than their parents.

Unfortunately, the establishment prefers to "cloak itself in ignorance." I don't mean to imply that the men and women of science are ignorant. Instead, I simply submit that the overwhelming empirical evidence discerned through observation should be enough to conclude that there is a relationship between specific habits, toxins, etc. and degenerative diseases. In a strange irony, science, the toolset relied upon for creating new knowledge, is actually a cloak of ignorance in complex systems like the human body. It draws out, over a long period of time, the discovery of truths that we already suspect.

I have often heard that the definition of insanity is doing the same thing over and over and expecting different results. If that is accurate, then it is insane to expect science to give us an understanding of human health in the short term. Science has done a tremendous amount to help us understand the physical world. We have high confidence in results that are scientifically valid, but the field of human health is too complex for science to give us answers that we feel confident about in time to save our species. We have to suspend the requirement for exactness in order to make progress in the field of health.

Science, and as an adjunct, medicine, will no doubt fight the notion of using a preponderance of the evidence instead of scientific proof for making decisions about human health. Maybe this approach is the wrong one to choose to follow, but I am 100% sure that waiting for science to mature is not the right one. To those who would fight against an alternative to scientific proof, know that daVinci also said, "Anyone who constructs an argument by appealing to authority is not using his intelligence. He is just using his memory."

Profit: The Chairman of the Board
In an article in *Experience Life Magazine* entitled "The New View of Health," writer, Kelly Grace wrote, "Healthcare consumers, providers and policy makers are waking up to the fact that conventional Western medicine with its dependence on long-term pharmaceutical use and expensive interventions – is not serving the real needs of a population (and economy) in the throes of a chronic disease crisis." In order to serve the needs of the population, many, like Kelly and I, believe that Western medicine must shift its emphasis from the treatment of sick people to the prevention of sickness in well people. We believe that it must shift from the treatment of symptoms found in those who are already sick to the implementation of habits, techniques, routines, etc. that can prevent the causes of sickness altogether.

Unfortunately, there is a financial motivation *not* to do that. Sick care is far easier to productize, and therefore profit from, than prevention. Billions and billions of dollars are at stake and, if you are in the medical industry, why would you want to change? Shareholders would suffer because it would be incredibly difficult for the entire industry to shift.

How could pharmaceutical companies that have billions invested in labs that research chemicals and factories that turn chemicals into pills, shots, inhalers, ointments, etc. productize something that doesn't involve chemicals without a fundamental shift and significant financial losses? How could doctors, heavily trained in diagnosing and managing trauma, disease and sickness and lacking training in fields like nutrition and exercise, help patients adopt preventive health habits? How could hospitals that generate the lion's share of their revenue from reactive care monetize proactive care? There would be an incredible impact on the profit of these organizations. And that is why I believe that *profit*, another of the cornerstones of Western civilization, along with its partner in crime, *science*, have abducted human health.

As you read above, I believe that science progresses too slowly in complex systems like the human body. And, I believe that for-profit business lacks the necessary "conscience" to consider that which is important to human health. This is because, at its core, for-profit business has only one instruction: to increase profit. Rain or shine, day or night, war or peace, hat-making or healthcare – increase profit. Weak or strong economy, good or bad product, happy or unhappy customers, hamburgers or hospital beds – increase profit. Every month, every quarter, every year – increase profit.

For-profit business lacks a "conscience" about human health because it forces businesses (and the people that operate within them) to make decisions based on a single criteria – will this decision increase profit? Of course, many of the people operating in the medical industry have made decisions that were good for human health *and* good for profit, but I submit that those are merely coincidences. Over time, the overwhelming majority of decisions in any for-profit business operating in a for-profit paradigm are made solely because they increase profit. These decisions may be bad for the employees (layoffs, benefit reductions, pay cuts), they may be bad for suppliers (competitive bidding, price renegotiation, offshore production) and they may be bad for consumers (price increases, product line changes, health and safety risks that are within the bounds of the law), but the decisions are always (suppose to be) good for shareholders because they are always intended to increase profit now or in the future. For-profit companies are just that: for-profit. And they are not *for* anything else, despite what the annual report says.

Hmm. I sound like a communist, don't I? Well, I'm not. I am a proud American. In fact, I am an engineer by education and an entrepreneur by profession. That makes me both a scientist and a capitalist. I believe in science as a discipline for the discovery and organization of facts and I think that for-profit capitalism is the social-economic-political paradigm that is best suited to the striving character of mankind. However, like all human inventions, both science and capitalism have limits. They both fail in certain situations.

Follow the Money
In the U.S., we spend more on health care per person (roughly $7,000 per year) and more as a percent of GDP (just over 16%) than any other country in the world. The gross domestic product of the United States is just over $13 trillion dollars and $2.1 trillion of that is spent on healthcare. By contrast, Americans spend $520 billion, or 4% of GDP, on food and beverages annually. The rising cost of treatment combined with longer, but more diseased life spans has resulted in the highest healthcare cost per person in the world.

As discussed earlier, for-profit companies are chartered to do whatever it takes (within the law) to make their profit grow. In general, this is the purpose of any for-profit business. By taking a closer look at one group of for-profit companies in the health care field, pharmaceutical companies, you can easily see that they are consistently *for* profit, and not necessarily *for* anything else.

Between 1994 and 2004, the U.S. population grew by 12%. Meanwhile, the number of prescriptions in the U.S. rose from 2.1 billion to 3.5 billion, a 68% increase. Incredibly, 24% of people under 18 take at least one prescription medication – 35% between the ages of 18 and 44, 62% between 45 and 64, and 84% of people over 65 take prescription drugs. However, the meteoric increase in the use of prescription drugs only tells part of the story. Drug prices are way up too.

Drug prices have increased an average of 8.3% annually since 1994 while inflation for that same time period was about 2.5% per year. Pharmaceutical companies typically blame their high prices on the exorbitant cost of bringing a drug to market. Without question, the U.S. Food and Drug Administration has a long and arduous approval process. And that explanation for high costs would stand up were it not for the fact that drug-making ranked as the third most profitable industry in the world, just behind crude oil production and commercial banking. Pharmaceutical companies have an average profit margin of 16% compared to the 5% median profit margin for all Fortune 500 companies. While the FDA drug approval process certainly drives some of the cost, it is clear that hefty profits do as well.

Drug companies are essentially chemistry labs with a marketing department. The scientists do research on common ailments and diseases - those that affect a large enough population to be a viable market - and create chemical combinations to try to reduce the symptoms or, occasionally the cause, of a "popular" ailment or disease. A successfully marketed drug can generate billions of dollars of revenue and profit for a pharmaceutical company. So, marketers work very hard to make sure that drugs get to market in a positive light. This profit motivation, combined with loose regulations, creates an atmosphere in which the public's health is a secondary consideration behind the primary consideration, which is profit growth.

The primary distributors of drugs in the United States are its roughly 700,300 doctors. Those doctors make treatment decisions for their patients based on supposedly objective, scientific information they learn in school, at medical conferences and in medical journals. In 2005 and 2006, the press uncovered that that (profit-motivated) pharmaceutical companies use these forums as marketing opportunities to influence doctor behavior for the distribution of their drugs. Below is a sampling of the discoveries:

- Vioxx, a painkiller made by Merck, was pulled off of the market in 2005 as a result of an increased risk of heart attack after 18 months of use. During the investigation, the *New England Journal of Medicine* (the most widely-read medical journal for doctors) reported that it had discovered that Merck had removed data from a 2000 Merck-sponsored study, printed in its journal, about three Vioxx users that suffered heart attacks.

- *The New England Journal of Medicine* later reported that companies including Merck, Pfizer and GlaxoSmithKline obscure information when reporting on drug trials. Some drug companies kept negative findings secret and only published positive results.

- A scientist hired by Proctor & Gamble to study its osteoporosis drug Actonel, a drug that generates over $1 billion annually, alleged that his findings were misrepresented by P&G and presented at several prominent medical meetings with doctors.

- *The Journal of Thoracic and Cardiovascular Surgery* revealed the financial ties between the scientific researchers that authored a study on a system to treat an abnormal heart rhythm and the manufacturer of that system, AtriCure, Inc. The researchers, well-known doctors at The Cleveland Clinic (a prominent heart center) and the University of Cincinnati, did not disclose their financial ties to the manufacturer when they published their study. Their financial ties included stock options, consulting contracts and royalty payments.

- Describing its turnaround plans, Merck & Co. said that it is instituting a "new commercial model" to get the message about its drugs to patients, doctors and health plans more efficiently. The new model involves hiring opinion leaders – leading doctors in particular disease categories – as consultants to influence other doctors.

So, let me review my comments about the pharmaceutical industry: it is large, fast growing, very profitable and, well, not necessarily driven by a commitment to human health. Should it surprise anyone that the pharmaceutical industry operates primarily in the interest of profit, commonly neglecting risks to human health? Probably not. "Grow profit" is the single over-arching charter of a for-profit company.

What is surprising, to me at least, are the attacks that the pharmaceutical industry, and its ally, The Food and Drug Administration, wage on competition (alternative medicine, as it has been labeled), regardless of the benefits that that competition may provide for human health. Attacks on competition are nothing new in free enterprise, but when one group can use its financial and regulatory leverage along with its stronghold on "legitimate" medicine to disrupt and destroy alternatives that have benefits to our species, something is terribly, terribly wrong.

Let me be clear here on my stance regarding so-called alternative medicine, lest you conclude that I have an agenda to promote that crowd. There are some (*some*) well-intentioned, well educated people in the field of alternative medicine and I believe that there is a lot to learn from them. I believe that those in the alternative medicine field have as much right to opine on human health as those in mainstream medicine and I believe that you and I should have unfiltered access to all legitimate information relating to the health or our species. Bottom line: I am strongly opposed to one field of health stifling the progress of another in the name of profit – and you should be too!

How would you feel if you found out that oil companies were using their financial and regulatory leverage in a coordinated effort to disrupt the progress of companies developing alternative energy sources? Mad, I hope. Well, this is the same thing!

Below, I have reprinted an article exactly as it appeared on www.cnn.com on February 22, 2006, that aptly demonstrates how the pharmaceutical industry uses the federal government and the irreproachable names of science and traditional medicine to undermine an effective, alternative therapy for arthritis in the pursuit of profit growth.

"Popular Supplements Do Little for Arthritis
Two hot-selling supplements used by millions of Americans are of little help to most people with mild arthritis, concludes a large government study that is part of an effort to scrutinize unregulated health remedies.

For most arthritis patients with aching knees, the health food store supplements, glucosamine and chondroitin sulfate, turned out to be no better than dummy pills. People who had more acute knee pain seemed to show some benefit.

Rheumatologist Dr. Daniel Clegg of the University of Utah in Salt Lake City, who led the study, suggested people with severe arthritis talk to their doctors about trying the supplements short-term to see if they work.

More than 20 million Americans suffer from osteoarthritis, the most common form of arthritis. That number is expected to double in the next two decades as baby boomers age. Osteoarthritis is a degenerative joint disease that affects the knees, hips, back and the small joints in the fingers.

The search for pain relief helped boost worldwide sales of glucosamine and chondroitin to $1.7 billion last year, according to the Nutrition Business Journal, which tracks supplements. The supplements -- made from animal cartilage and shellfish -- have had even wider appeal amid safety concerns over certain painkillers, including the arthritis medicine Vioxx, which was yanked from the market in 2004.

At least 5 million Americans use the two supplements either alone or together, government figures show. President Bush was among the customers for a while because of knee pain, but spokeswoman Dana Perino said Wednesday the president no longer takes the supplements. Bush has replaced running with mountain biking.

The supplements showed no known side effects during the government's six-month study, but the scientists didn't address the safety of longer-term use.

The arthritis research, published in Thursday's New England Journal of Medicine, is the third major study in a year to find no overall benefit from some of the most popular nutritional supplements. Recently, research showed the herb saw palmetto didn't reduce symptoms of an enlarged prostate, and last year a study indicated Echinacea didn't prevent or treat colds.

Unlike drugs, such supplements are not regulated by the U.S. Food and Drug Administration and their makers don't have to prove the products are safe or effective.

The Arthritis Foundation said Wednesday it was recommending people with severe knee pain speak to their doctors about whether combined glucosamine-chondroitin therapy might be a good addition to their overall treatment. Generally, arthritis sufferers are urged to exercise, keep their weight down and try hot and cold therapy, along with painkillers if needed.

One person who plans to keep using the supplements is 72-year-old Irene Schwartzburt. She said the unregulated remedies relieved the "sticking pain" in her right knee when painkillers failed.

"I want to stay active," said the retired teacher from Plainview, New York. "The supplements work for me so why not continue with them?"

In the government study, funded by the National Institutes of Health, 1,583 patients with arthritis knee pain received one of five treatments: either glucosamine or chondroitin, a combination of both, the painkiller Celebrex or dummy pills. Neither the doctors nor patients knew which treatment was given.

After six months, patients filled out a questionnaire to determine how many felt a 20 percent reduction in pain. Researchers found the supplements when taken alone or together were no more effective than dummy pills at pain relief.

Sixty percent who took the dummy medication had reduced pain compared with 64 percent who took glucosamine, 65 percent who took chondroitin and 67 percent who took the combo pills. These differences were so small that they could have occurred by chance alone.

The drug Celebrex did reduce pain -- 70 percent reported improvement -- affirming the study's validity. However, the drug is being studied to see if it's safe for people at risk of heart problems.

Of the 354 people with moderate to severe pain, 79 percent who took both supplements reported relief compared with 54 percent who took the dummy pills and 69 percent who took Celebrex.
In a journal editorial, Dr. Marc Hochberg of the University of Maryland noted the study's limitations: a high dropout rate (20 percent) and a whopping 60 percent who said the dummy pills made them feel better -- double the usual placebo effect. Hochberg has received consulting fees from Pfizer Inc., which makes Celebrex, and Merck & Co., which made Vioxx.

Clegg and 10 other researchers in the study reported receiving fees or grant support from Pfizer or McNeil Consumer & Specialty Pharmaceuticals, which makes Tylenol.

The Council for Responsible Nutrition, which represents dietary supplement makers, said it was pleased about the positive findings in the severe arthritis group."

Now that you have read the article, ask yourself the following questions:

1. Compare the statements surrounding the result that 67% had reduced pain when taking glucosamine and chondroitin ("These differences were so small that they could have occurred by chance alone") to the statements surrounding the result that 70% had reduced pain when taking Celebrex ("...affirming the study's validity"). Does the article appear to attack glucosamine and chondroitin as ineffective and declare Celebrex as effective when only three percentage points separate them in the overall study?

2. Did you notice that 79% of people with moderate to severe pain reported relief with glucosamine and chondroitin, while only 69% of people with moderate to severe pain reported relief with Celebrex? Does it feel as if the authors buried that piece of data?

3. Does the headline match the content of the article?

4. Why include references to inconclusive research on the herbs saw palmetto and Echinacea when they have nothing to do with arthritis? Why imply that there might be long-term side effects to glucosamine and chondroitin when there is no evidence of this?

5. Do you believe that doctors who receive consulting fees from drug makers and write articles are objective?

6. Do you think that the CEO of Pfizer, the maker of Celebrex, considers glucosamine and chondroitin to be serious competition given that they are used by 25% of his potential consumers (5 million of 20 million arthritis sufferers)? Do you think he is motivated to undermine the public's confidence in glucosamine and chondroitin?

To be sure, there are a lot of quacks out to make a fast buck espousing false health claims about the next wonder plant and praying on the fears and dreams of people and we have to protect the public from them. However, that is the job of government, not the medical industry.

To lump all alternatives into the category of quackery as the article above tries to do is itself quackery, or worse. For mainstream medicine, specifically the pharmaceutical industry, to protect its profit interests by attacking and discrediting legitimate, alternative solutions to human health problems proves only one thing: it *is* all about the money.

And, in reality, medicines derived organically are probably more effective and safer than chemically-derived medicines because organically-based medicines are more complete in their chemical and biological makeup. They are probably less foreign to the human "organism" because of their complete chemical and biological makeup (synthetic medicines are chemicals produced in isolation). They originated and developed alongside the plants and animals (including us) on this planet whereas chemically-derived drugs were invented by scientists in a lab. Plants and animals endured together, sharing the same environment for thousands of years, and, therefore, are more apt to assimilate to one another.

As this article so clearly demonstrates, the profit motive leverages the irreproachable name of science to abduct health. It shows how pharmaceutical companies work to change public perception about an alternative to their productized synthetic drugs in an effort to shift consumer perceptions and spending. These moves are not made in the name of health. They are done in the name of profit.

In pursuit of profit growth, companies attack competition. However, when, in the name of profit growth, the pharmaceutical industry, or any industry, actively works to deceive people about options that may improve their health, it is a *crime against humanity*. As I said earlier, I believe in science and for-profit business. But, as creations of man, each has its limitations. And, this is the exact place where the profit motive reaches its limit. With its single, universal command to increase profit – every day, every month, every quarter – capitalism, as a social-political-economic framework, lacks the "conscience" necessary to protect our species (and our planet).

From Sick Care to Prevention
The pharmaceutical industry has endured its share of attacks over the last decade or so and has, in many ways, become the whipping post for the failure of modern medicine. I join those whipping on the pharmaceutical industry not because I believe that it is the axis of evil in healthcare, but

because it is the best example of how for-profit business fails to consider collateral damage as it operates *for-profit* and not *for anything else.*

In a for-profit business, managers are required to invest the resources of their company in endeavors that will increase the profit of their companies. More and more evidence suggests that most degenerative diseases and chronic illness are a result of the cumulative effect of our lifestyle choices. But changing lifestyle choices is not something that the healthcare industry is suited to profit from. Medicines, and more specifically drugs, target the symptoms of illness because symptoms are usually easier for the healthcare industry to isolate and treat than the cause of an illness. However, for you and me, symptoms are also what create discomfort and we are willing to pay to relieve discomfort. So, healthcare is more equipped to treat symptoms and we are more than willing to pay to relieve the discomfort that comes from them. As a result, we see dozens of new and improved sick-care treatments hitting the market and comparatively little in the area of sickness prevention.

This makes sense if you are a shareholder. However, it makes no sense if you are a human being. Consider this analogy: If you went home today and noticed that the wood on your house had suddenly become pitted, dusty and weak, would you call a carpenter to replace the wood or would you call a pest control company to deal with the termites that have obviously been feasting on your house? Calling a carpenter to replace your house's pitted, weakened wood would address the symptom, but replacing the wood only provides more of a meal for the little pests. Replacing the wood and expecting the termites to go away would be madness, right? Eventually, your house would become so weak that it would fall in on itself.

However, if 99% of the homeowners with termite problems called a carpenter and paid them to replace their wood instead of calling a pest control service to kill the termites, guess how many carpenters and how many termite control services there would be? Guess who would dominate the yellow pages under "TERMITE?" Carpenters. Because all of the money for termite problems would flow to carpenters, there would not be many termite-focused pest control services. But people are not that foolish, right?

Unfortunately, this is exactly what happens in healthcare. When we get sick, we go see someone in the healthcare industry that often recommends or prescribes some type of symptom alleviating drug, therapy or surgery, and often nothing is done about the underlying cause of the sickness – their lifestyles and habits. We continue to get sick and we continue to pay the medical industry over and over again for drug-centered treatments to address the symptoms of our illness, largely ignoring that which is causing it (the termites keep coming back and we keep calling a carpenter). This cycle repeats itself, very profitably for the medical industry I might add, until eventually, we get some serious chronic illness, degenerate and die (our house falls in on itself).

As a result of the flow of money and profit, the healthcare "yellow pages" is dominated by treatment and we see very little prevention. For-profit healthcare will continue to pour its resources into treating symptoms as long as that is where we spend our money.

I am not optimistic that government can (or should) effectively regulate capitalism to have a conscience. And I do not believe that we will make healthcare non-profit. Free enterprise in healthcare has too many benefits and too much support for that to happen. However, I believe, as you will read, that we can shift from a focus on sick-care to a focus on prevention by leveraging the profit motive itself.

In a free enterprise, capitalist economy, everything starts and ends with *how you spend your money*. Because of this, I believe that the change we need, from an emphasis on sick-care to an emphasis on sickness prevention, can result if people become educated about human health and change how they spend their money. We can use the profit motive to our advantage, changing our lifestyle habits, and therefore our spending habits and the profit zombies (either the companies that exist now or those that will move into the void) will shift their direction, pouring their abundant resources into sickness prevention.

We, the Consumers
After spending over $2 trillion ($2,000,000,000,000) per year in health care over the last 10 or so years, deaths from heart disease, cancer and stroke – the nation's three leading killers – are down only 1% to 3%. Think about that for a second. In the last decade, we've spent over $20 trillion – almost twice the gross national product of the U.S. – and we haven't made a dent in the nation's three leading killers!

How could anyone argue that the current approach to healthcare is working? Healthcare has failed to care for our health. The evidence is overwhelming. With mountains of money spent and very little improvement in death rates from the nation's top killers, it is clear that we are not caring for health, but merely treating sickness.

To improve the health or our species, we have to change the entire healthcare system. Before you roll your eyes, know that changing the healthcare system is not that hard. It doesn't require a large, well-funded study. It doesn't require letters to your congressman or a march on Washington. It doesn't require congressional hearings. In fact, it doesn't require any government intervention at all. It only requires you to change the way you spend your money.

We, the consumers (the spenders of money), are the ones who direct all for-profit industries including the healthcare industry. For-profit businesses are like machines with but one simple instruction: grow profit. The profit machine will follow its profit imperative like a bloodhound after an escaped convict. As long as you and I prioritize comfort over cause, as long as we are willing to continue to settle for the relief of discomfort over the elimination and prevention of the root causes of disease, the healthcare industry is compelled by its profit imperative to oblige you.

We could do a lot with $20 trillion.

Chapter 3

The Cumulative Effect

Health is not simply the absence of sickness.

Hannah Greene

A Glimpse of our Future
Somewheretown, USA, the year 2025

Everywhere you go, from Walgreens to Wal*Mart, from the magazine rack to the men's room, society revolves around sick care. Angioplasty to unblock clogged arteries is as common as a colonoscopy. Senility and Alzheimer's is almost a certainty for those unlucky enough to live past 75. There is a near 100% chance of developing cancer. Wal*Mart has one-fourth of its parking lot dedicated to the handicapped and they provide nearly as many motorized shopping carts as push shopping carts. Medicine accounts for one out of every four dollars of GNP and 40% of the square footage of the average grocery store. At the checkout, the magazine racks are filled with a new type of lifestyle magazine – those devoted to individual diseases (Type II Digest, Full Figure, Cardio Rhythms, etc.). There is nearly 50% obesity and the locals choose buffet-style restaurants and wear giant, baggy sweat clothes. There are entire stores devoted to tobacco and football field-sized liquor stores. New construction is dominated by healthcare. The average adult over 55 takes 8-12 prescription pills per day and the national conversation is dominated by illness instead of progress, national pride and… living.

The expected lifespan of an American has increased over 20% in 65 years due to advances in medicine. According to the Social Security Administration, the life expectancy of an American born in 1940 was 63.6 years and the life expectancy of an American born in 2004 was 77.3 years. Modern medicine successfully treats many injuries, infections, bacteria and viruses that would have easily killed us years ago. In addition, treatments continually emerge that extend the lives of those afflicted with disease.

The data has shown that we are, indeed, living longer, but aren't we really living longer, sicker? Aren't we living longer because of infection treatment, trauma care and disease management, not because we are healthier? Would our average lifespan decrease if we compared apples to apples? If we eliminated trauma care, infection treatment and disease management and rolled medicine back to the way it was 70 years ago, do you think our life expectancy would be longer or shorter today than the 63.6 years that it was in 1940? In other words, if you take out advances in reactionary sick care and trauma care, if medicine was exactly as it was 70 years ago, do you think we would be living longer or shorter lives than we did in 1940?

Don't worry about venturing a guess. The question has already been answered, in my view. In March, 2005, *The New England Journal of Medicine* reported that, for the first time in history, the current generation of children is expected to have a shorter life expectancy than their parents. The effects of obesity-related diseases like diabetes and heart disease along with lifestyle-related illnesses like cancer are expected to more than offset gains from medical advances over the next few decades. In other words, our sickness is outpacing our advances in medicine and many of the advances we've made over the last 70 years. People are so sick today that the advances in sick care that added nearly 14 years to the average American's lifespan can no longer sustain human health for the benchmark that was set in 2004.

The D-Generation
Jordan Rubin, author of "The Maker's Diet" observed that people born in the early 20th century, the World War II generation, suffer(ed) from diseases of old age like Alzheimer's, Osteoporosis, dementia and senility. People born in the Baby Boom generation of the 1940's and 1950's are the generation of obesity-related heart disease, stroke and cancer. Generation X-ers and Y-ers, those born in the 1980's and 1990's, are the first generation of young people to suffer such an alarming rate of autoimmune diseases like lupus, Crohn's disease and Type I diabetes. Looking at the trend lines on chronic illnesses, it seems clear that people born in the 21st century are doomed to suffer from all of these awful

degenerative illnesses. This is the generation of *degeneration*. This is the D-generation.

Normal lifespan begins at birth and lasts as long as the body can sustain life. Life is sustained because cells divide and regenerate tissue. However, there is a natural limit to the number of times cells can divide. This limit is called the Hayflick limit. When cells hit this limit, they cease to be able to divide and regenerate tissue and they have reached what scientists call senescence. Skin cells, for example, reach senescence before other parts of the body and cease producing new skin cells and that is why older people have thin, inelastic, wrinkled skin.

When cells stop reproducing, age-related illnesses can set in. Living a healthy life, therefore, means living a life free of chronic disease until some age-related illness brought on by senescence eventually kills you. In other words, a healthy person is someone who is free from sickness and disease until he becomes ill and dies from senescence (or dies from accidental death).

Many of us will not be fortunate enough to die from age-related illness. For many of us, a force will act on us (what I refer to later as the Cumulative Effect) to impact our bodies' regenerative abilities inside of our normal lifespan and it will either shorten our lifespan or reduce the quality of our remaining life. Very simply put, when genes are damaged by free radicals, chemical toxins, etc., and the cell divides before the gene damage can be repaired, daughter cells are born with genetic damage and – in an environment where the immune system is not functioning properly – these genetic damages accumulate and can lead to chronic illness and disease.

We're So Modern
Those of us living in developed countries, especially America, are raised to believe that we are among the most fortunate people in the world. However, life expectancy in America ranks 42nd worldwide, down from 11th two decades ago. Those people living in primitive agricultural societies are far healthier than those living on the modern diet of developed countries. Primitive cultures, living the way our ancestors did, rarely die of diet, habit, and lifestyle-related diseases primarily because they eat healthier and have more active lifestyles. Primitive cultures eat to live whereas modern cultures live to eat. In our modern culture, we live

for convenience and pleasure, doing and eating things that are easy and feel good. In the harsh light of truth, the diet of the developed world may be the only thing that has actually gotten worse as the rest of our lives have gotten better over the last several centuries.

Jordan Rubin estimates that our ancestors got 30 to 65 percent of their daily calories (and up to 100 grams of fiber a day) from vegetables and fruit. Today that is hardly the case. In developed countries, we get the majority of our calories from meat, fat, simple sugar and refined grains.

An average American man will wake up at 6:00 a.m. after six to seven hours of sleep, shower and prepare for work. He will likely eat a pastry and drink coffee as he drives to work (refined flour, high fructose corn syrup, hydrogenated fat, caffeinated coffee sprayed with pesticides). Then, he'll sit virtually motionless at his desk and during meetings for hours. Later, he will probably drive to lunch and order a sandwich with chips or a burger with fries and a diet soda (antibiotic-treated, pesticide-fed meat, pesticide-grown lettuce and tomato on refined flour roll with polyunsaturated fat and trans fat-laden mayonnaise and fries or chips, chemical-rich city water mixed with aspartame-containing caffeinated diet soda). After lunch, he'll drive back to his office and sit at his desk and in meetings for several more hours. He will probably get hungry again before the end of the day so he'll wander over to the snack machine and get something like cheese crackers and a diet soda for a snack (sodium and polyunsaturated-fat laden processed cheese crackers and an aspartame-containing caffeinated diet soda that has leached aluminum from its can). At the end of his work day, he'll drive home worrying about today's problems and tomorrow's work. He'll greet his family; eat a traditional American dinner like spaghetti (simple-sugar-rich pasta with antibiotic-treated, pesticide-fed ground beef and sodium-rich tomato sauce, refined flour garlic bread with trans-fat containing margarine) and have a glass or two of beer. He'll end his day sitting on his couch, watching two hours of news programs on television or reading the news of the day, then go to bed between 11:00 PM and midnight.

What is wrong with this picture? No exercise, no water, no fruit (maybe a blueberry or two in the morning pastry), no vegetables (save a piece of iceberg lettuce on the lunch sandwich which does not have much in the way of nutritional value, a slice of tomato and some tomato sauce), and no grains. Lots of caffeine, a good bit of simple sugar, some alcohol, a lot of exposure to chemical toxins (water in fountain soda, antibiotics and pesticides in the meat, pesticides residue on lettuce and tomato, aspartame in the diet soda and myriad toxins in the city water mixed into his diet soda), too little sleep, too much stress and a lot of free radical forming polyunsaturated fats and trans-fats.

One day like this or even one week following these habits would not be so bad, but we have entire nations of people who follow a regimen like this (and far worse) for decades and then they wonder why they have become sick. What do you think happens to your body when you follow this routine for 11,000 days (30 years)? The body regenerates and replaces nearly all of its cells every year. How can you expect your body to reproduce healthy cells when you do not provide it with the nutrition that it needs? Imagine repeating the above routine 11,000 times. Can you honestly expect that you would be a healthy person?

In the last thousand years, the whole world has advanced – shelter, energy, transportation, communication, etc. – allowing a significant improvement in comfort, convenience and lifestyle. However, I submit that one thing in our society which has gone backwards in the last thousand years is our health. Sure, we are living longer, but don't be fooled by the propaganda. We are living longer thanks to advances in trauma care, infectious disease vaccines and chemical and surgical intervention, but we are increasingly sick and degenerated. Drugs and trauma care keep us alive longer, but what kind of existence is it? We're sick, degenerated, fat, arthritic, frail, senile people. We're living longer, but we're not living better. We chemically and surgically intervene to prolong life, but the life that is left is one of poor health and suffering.

I believe that there are four major trends that act in combination with our individual genetic predisposition to certain diseases to impact health as we age. First, we now consume more toxins and significantly more unhealthy food than ever before. This is because we have a polluted water supply, an array of harmful food toxins like pesticides and hormones in use, thousands of environmental pollutants in contact with humans, an abundance of fat and simple sugar in the modern diet and an overuse of tobacco, alcohol, caffeine, and pharmaceutical drugs.

Second, the food we do eat has far less nutrition in it than it had in the past. Volume farming methods do not adequately replenish the soil, resulting in significantly less nutrient content in most of the fruits and vegetables grown today and food processing strips most of the remaining nutritional content out of the packaged foods that make up much of the modern diet.

Third, people in developed countries eat more calories. This is because their diets are built around calorie-dense foods like meat, portion sizes are larger than ever, and there is a nearly ubiquitous availability of packaged, convenience food. And fourth, as man has progressed, he has made his life more convenient. Transportation is almost completely automated, many modern jobs involve zero manual labor and technologies such as television and the computer make life more sedentary. These four trends combine to create an increasingly unhealthy lifestyle for the modern man or woman and accumulate health consequences as we age.

As a result of these trends, chronic illness has become incredibly common and we seem to accept it as a normal part of aging. But chronic illness simply isn't a natural part of aging. Retirement? Convalescent homes? Walkers and wheelchairs? How often have you read about "retired people" or "old folk's homes" from any period in history before the late-1900's? People didn't retire. They didn't go into assisted living facilities – they worked their whole lives. In order to do that, they had to be healthy. Our ancestors truly went from cradle to school to work to grave. Today, people in developed countries go from cradle to school to work to retirement to cradle to grave. And in the not-too-distant future, I believe that the D-generation will go from cradle to school to work to cradle to grave, succumbing to chronic illness before even reaching retirement.

Harmony

Sixty-five million years ago in what is now the Yucatan Peninsula (in Southeastern Mexico), it is believed that an event took place that suddenly and dramatically changed the earth's environment. Geologists believe that a meteor impacted the earth, throwing huge amounts of matter into the atmosphere. This event is believed to have created months of darkness and much cooler temperatures globally, and the resulting harsh conditions led to the extinction of many species, including the last of the dinosaurs. The plants and animals that had slowly adapted to survive in the climate that existed just prior to the impact of the meteor were no longer able to survive in a suddenly colder climate. In other words, when the environment of the earth changed, species that were not suited for the new environment, and those that could not adapt fast enough, died off. When species are unable to adapt to their environment and die off like this, it is often referred to as *natural selection*.

About 75 years ago, the Hoover dam was built in the middle of the Arizona desert. Prior to that time, the Pima Indians that lived in the area were a healthy Indian tribe that stretched from Arizona to Mexico. They subsisted by farming their own fruits and vegetables. However, when the U.S. government built the Hoover Dam, the Pima in Arizona could no longer irrigate their crops. So the government provided food for them, but the government-provided food was substantially different than what they had eaten in the past. This food was the standard American fare – rife with fat, stripped of nutrients and dense with calories.

Today, the Pima in Arizona are among the most obese groups of people in the world and they have the highest prevalence of type 2 diabetes on Earth (exceeding 50% of adults, much more than is observed in other U.S. populations). The increased diabetes prevalence is likely a result of a sudden shift in diet from traditional agricultural goods to man-made, processed foods. For comparison, genetically similar Pimas in Mexico continue to live as they always have and they have virtually no type 2 diabetes (affecting less than 4%).

So, what do a meteor and The Hoover Dam have to do with one another? Each changed the environment of living species, triggering a form of natural selection on those species affected.

The life forms on our planet thrive in a state of biological stability and they either adapt or die off when their environment changes. That is, all life forms on earth seek to live in harmony with their surroundings and, scientists maintain, have adaptive mechanisms that help them try to achieve this harmony when their environment changes. History shows us that some species can adapt and some species cannot. Scientists believe that success depends on the magnitude of the adaptation needed to survive. In all cases, the period of adaptation is a challenging one for the species as it is living out of harmony with its environment.

And even with this adaptation capability apparently native to all life forms, when harmony is achieved, history shows us that it appears to be relatively delicate. Ecosystems can be easily disturbed by invading organisms, plants, animals, chemicals and weather changes. Like a church choir singing together for the first time, harmony is hard to achieve and easy to disrupt.

For the Pima Indians in Arizona, the Hoover Dam might as well have been a meteor. In about 1932, the delicate harmony that the tribe had achieved with its environment over hundreds and hundreds of years suddenly and dramatically changed. Their diets had been built around plant foods and they lived active lives farming crops and then, quite suddenly, they were sedentary and eating a diet built around processed foods.

When something disrupts the delicate balance and persists, the system, which achieved its balance very slowly, adjusts slowly. When one singer in the choir gets out of harmony and stays there, the rest of the group cannot quickly adjust to bring everyone back into harmony. Instead, the system becomes unbalanced and begins to break down.

Over the last sixty to seventy years, I believe that the developed world has undergone a significant change, altering the environment for the humans living in it, and we are experiencing the challenges of being out of harmony with our environment (showing up as epidemic levels of chronic illness). Although not as dramatic as the impact of a meteor, I believe that the resulting change has substantially altered the environment for all species, including our own. I call this environmental change the *Synthetic Shift* and, this time, the human race is the source of the change – not a meteor.

The Synthetic Shift is the result of the tens of thousands of man-made chemicals that have been introduced into earth's delicate ecosystem since the end of World War II in combination with the dramatic change in the diet and lifestyle of people living in developed countries. The environment in which our species lives – the air we breathe, the water we drink, the food we eat, the way we work, sleep and rest – has substantially changed in the last several decades. Although not as sudden or as dramatic as the impact of a meteor, the Synthetic Shift has changed, and will continue to change, the environment in which man lives in ways that are profound and maybe permanent for all life forms.

As biochemical organisms, humans achieved harmony with their environment. The proof is that our species is still alive. Over thousands of years, the process of natural selection killed everything off that did not adapt and achieve harmony with its surroundings.

Nature doesn't know how to protect itself. This is the job of natural selection. It is said of natural selection that, with time, the fox and the rabbit both get faster. The foxes catch the slow rabbits before they are able to reproduce. So, only the fast rabbits reproduce, passing on the speedy gene to their offspring. Then the slower foxes can't catch the fast rabbits so they, too, die off young, leaving only the fast foxes to reproduce and pass on the speedy gene. This is how natural selection happens and helps a species adapt.

In the 19th and 20th century in the developed and developing world, when man moved from the field to the factory to the office, his lifestyle changed considerably. He was far more sedentary than he had ever been at any point in the history of the species. Then, beginning in the mid-20th century, he began to mass-produce processed foods and beverages, changing the nutrition content of his diet more significantly than at any point in the history of the species. And if that wasn't enough change, at about the same time, he began to create and produce thousands and thousands of new chemicals for common use that had never been encountered by the species at any point in history. These chemicals were frequently encountered by man in everything from crop fertilization and cleaning products to food additives and foot creams.

The changes were radical and it seems man's harmony with his environment was disrupted. By introducing tens of thousands of chemical toxins, dramatically changing our eating, activity habits and lifestyles, we have changed the environment with which our species has reached a natural harmony. We have radically changed the "environment" that our bodies have developed to expect and the result is a sort of shock.

When the environment changes, species either evolve to adapt to it or they are naturally selected out. As I said above, the period when the species is working to adapt to its new surroundings is a challenging one for the species because it is living out of harmony with its environment. I believe that the epidemic of "unexplained" degenerative disease and chronic illness is evidence that we are experiencing the challenges of adapting to our new environment. I believe that we are seeing natural selection at work on the human race.

For years, the brightest financial minds in the world have tried to build models to predict the stock market's movements. The ability to accurately predict the movements of one or more financial markets would give the model's owner an advantage over every other person and firm trading, legally yielding the model's owner an incredible fortune. Alas, no one has ever been able to build such a model because the millions of variables that influence the overall market make it impossible to exactly replicate.

Similarly, meteorologists have been trying to build models of the earth's atmosphere for many years in order to accurately predict the weather, but we have all experienced the accuracy of meteorological forecasts. Accurate weather predictions are valuable for anybody living in the path of severe weather and for an array of businesses from farming to professional sports leagues to car washes. Like the financial markets, there are a vast number of variables that influence the weather. Not only are there millions of variables, but many of the variables influence one another (like heat and pressure). Modeling millions upon millions of combinations of variables, all interacting with one another, is beyond our current skill set.

Building models that can accurately predict complex systems is challenging, and I submit that there is an even more complex system than either the financial markets or the earth's atmosphere - the human body. The influences at work in and on the human body are vast: thousands of environmental factors, an incredibly diverse array of diet options, exposure to tens of thousands of different toxins, level of stress, air quality, amount and type of exercise, duration and quality of sleep, emotional health, vast genetic diversity, and the list goes on and on and on. As you might guess, if we can't yet build a model for financial markets or our atmosphere, we certainly can't yet build a model that can accurately predict the body's actions and reactions to its many influences.

The human body is like a puzzle with a billion pieces that we don't yet understand how to fit together. Does secondhand smoke cause breast cancer? How about French fries? Are pesticides neuro-toxic to humans? Is saturated fat good for me now? Do supplements improve health? Is aluminum linked to Alzheimer's? Is soy good or bad? Is genetically modified food dangerous? Why can't science say with certainty what causes cancer or arthritis or Attention Deficit Disorder or Parkinson's disease? Is this new piece of information a piece of the puzzle or is it the result of inter-relation of other pieces known or unknown?

It is comforting to think that someone, somewhere really has all of the answers about the human body. The truth, however uncomfortable it is for us to hear, is that we are still very primitive in our understanding of human health. We simply don't yet understand the complexities of the human body. Science has a very immature understanding of all of its intricacies (biological, chemical, emotional, spiritual, etc.). It is hard to believe that we could still be so primitive, but all the evidence one needs to conclude that the scientific-medical community does not understand the human body is the almost amusing lists of side effects associated with pharmaceutical drugs. With a complete understanding of the human body, scientists would be able to custom design molecules and combine them into drugs that did not create unintended "side" effects. It seems clear to me that the 30-40 potential side effects associated with the average drug is conclusive evidence enough to show that what we don't know about the human body far exceeds what we do know.

As a result of its largely incomplete understanding, medical science can't say with any certainty what causes many of the human body's problems and, worse, it cannot tell us how to fix them. Let's use my friend's understanding of computers as an analogy. My friend has very little understanding of how her computer actually works. She doesn't understand very much about the hardware or the software on her computer. She knows how to turn on the machine, launch a browser, and open her e-mail. She can deal with standard errors and make sure the mouse is plugged in, but if she encounters any real problems with the system, she is at a complete loss to diagnose the cause of the problem and fix it. My friend has had a computer for many years and, when she got it, she learned the basics relatively quickly. But her rate of learning new things about her computer since then has been very slow. Because she is not one to ask for help, she is learning her computer through discovery all on her own.

Medical science's understanding of the human body is near my friend's understanding of her computer. What medical science doesn't know about the human body exceeds what it does know today. It can address some of the basic problems effectively – trauma and infection, for example – but when it comes up against more challenging problems – neurological disorders like Alzheimer's or a molecular disease like cancer

— it is at a loss to diagnose the cause of the problem and fix it. And, like my friend, medical science's knowledge is improving, but it is incredibly slow. For now, the best medical science can do is figure this billion-piece puzzle out one piece at a time. Every time the medical community gets a breakthrough, we get a piece of the puzzle: cruciferous vegetables, fiber, hydrogenated fat, second-hand smoke, phytonutrients... puzzle piece, puzzle piece, puzzle piece.

Some day, we will have the entire puzzle put together and we will have a perfect view of cause and effect in the human body. Because we will know what causes diseases, we will be well equipped to cure them. Unfortunately, for now, medicine finds one piece here and there and sometimes gets a big breakthrough and puts together a whole section of puzzle pieces.

Until the day arrives when medicine has a complete or near-complete model of the human body, however, we are in a challenging position. We can continue to put our faith into a medical system that is based on fixing us when we break, but, try as it may, does not have the knowledge to fix most of what gets broken in us. Or, we can look at what is making sick people sick and try to prevent them from getting sick in the first place.

Sickness Misunderstood
Before we understood the geology of our planet, there were many theories about what caused earthquakes. In India, it was believed that the Earth was held up by four elephants that stood on the back of a turtle, which balanced on top of a cobra, and when any of these animals moved, the Earth trembled. According to Aristotle and the Greeks, earthquakes were caused by strong, wild winds trapped and held in caverns under the ground struggling to escape. And in Mozambique, it was believed that the earth was a living creature with the same kinds of problems people have, including getting sick with fever and chills, which we felt as the earth shaking.

This is all humorous now that we know what causes earthquakes, but it is evidence that, throughout history, we humans have proven that we won't sit around and wait for the facts. Instead, we tend to fill in the blanks with the theories that we think are most likely to become the truth. Worse, until the truth does become known, we accept the theories as truth.

This has happened with human health and several well-traveled myths have emerged. For example, many people believe that degenerative diseases like cancer simply happen to us. I call this the *spontaneous-disease myth*. Some unlucky mix of genetics and an unfortunate exposure to carcinogens causes people to win the cancer lottery, so to speak. As a result, people will often say that they or someone they know "got" cancer, arthritis, heart disease, etc. In reality, it really is more accurate to say that someone "developed" cancer, arthritis or heart disease because you don't "get" degenerative diseases. To say you "get" cancer or "get" arthritis or "get" heart disease implies spontaneity. In reality, we know that degenerative diseases happen to you slowly. Your body deteriorates until the weakened conditions exist that allow the disease to start.

To hear someone say, "Earl got cancer" or "Andy got arthritis" can also imply that something happened to them – like they caught something. You can "get" the flu because you can catch the flu bug, but you don't "get" cancer. There is no arthritis bug or heart disease bug or dementia bug. Degenerative diseases are largely self-inflicted. They are literally the cumulative result of the self-destructive choices that we make, mostly unaware that we are making them.

Another health myth is embodied in the oft-used statement, "Well... it finally caught up with him." Often, I hear people say this when they are referring to a sick or deceased friend or relative that maintained obviously bad habits over the years. I call this the *Tom & Jerry myth*. Like the cartoon Tom & Jerry, it is as if the disease (the cat) was chasing this person (the mouse), but the person had avoided capture countless times. But that is not what happened at all. Disease doesn't finally capture you after many narrow escapes. It grows inside of you. Little by little, drink by drink, bite by bite, belt hole by belt hole, pill by pill, day by sedentary day, disease accumulates in your body until it overpowers your weakened defenses.

Another myth about human health is what I call the *odd-and-unrelated-illness myth*. Cancer and other diseases are often found as a result of visiting a doctor about another health problem. So many times, I have heard, "The doctor found a lump/spot/blockage/mass when I went in to see him about my gall bladder/kidney stones/ emphysema/ blood pressure, etc." I have also heard many people report, "If I hadn't had shingles/ back spasms/ arthritis/ constipation/ whatever, the doctor would never have found my cancer/heart disease/liver disease, etc."

It is possible that multiple, unrelated health problems coincide in people, but as often as I have heard of this happening, it is not likely. The reality is, more often than not, much of the sickness and disease that people encounter together are actually resulting from the same cause. When the body is degenerated, it will simultaneously "malfunction" in many ways and in many areas because all of its systems support one another.

What is Really Happening
Not long ago, my wife deployed me an hour early to my daughter's school play to hold a half row of seats hostage. As I sat waiting alone in the auditorium for 45 minutes (men, some things are better left unsaid), I reached into my pocket and pulled out the change I had. In an effort to find something to pass the time, I decided to have a closer look at the change that I held in my hand. To my surprise, and for some reason it always surprises me, I found a quarter from 1970, the year I was born.

This quarter had seen a lot of action and had a lot of wear and tear. George Washington's face was worn and you could barely make out his features. There were chips and dents all over it and even the grooves around the edge of the coin were nearly smooth from decades of use. As I looked at the quarter, it occurred to me that this is how the average person's health must "look" at my age. A quarter has a tough life and, really, so do we humans.

At the most basic level, human health depends upon the reproduction of healthy cells and an effective immune system to ward off sickness. Both of these basic human health functions are severely impacted by the modern lifestyle. As stated earlier, there are several major human trends that have impacted human health.

Is it possible that the modern lifestyle in the west creates an accumulation of wear and tear on health like the accumulation of wear and tear on the quarter? If someone looked at you and all they could see was your health, would your health look like that quarter? Some interesting studies shed some light on these questions.

Dr. Weston Price, a Harvard-educated dentist, studied the nutritional habits of various primitive and advanced cultures on five continents during the 1930's in an effort to understand more about the causes of physical deformities that he saw as a dentist. He believed that dental health was an indicator of physical health and speculated that nutrition was to blame for the dental problems that he saw so frequently. Dr. Price and his wife sought out isolated, primitive cultures and compared their diet and dental health with those of advanced, mainstream societies.

The Prices found that people in primitive, isolated societies hunted, gathered and grew what they ate. None of the food they consumed was processed or refined and vegetables and fruit were often eaten raw. They also found that people in these societies had healthy, straight teeth and dental abnormalities were extremely rare. In contrast, those people living in modern societies had diets consisting largely of processed, cooked food that was high in salt, refined flour or sugar. Members of modern societies had crowded, crooked teeth, a great deal of tooth decay, and deformed jaws and dental arches were common.

Dr. Price concluded that the dental deformities in advanced societies were caused by the physical degeneration of the body resulting from poor nutrition. In 1939, Dr. Price published a paper entitled "Nutrition and Physical Degeneration" documenting his findings. Soon, medical doctors became involved in the study and, over time, they were able to document the introduction and rapid increase of degenerative diseases like cancer, heart disease, arthritis and diabetes as primitive societies adopted the habits of modern societies.

Dr. Dennis Burkett, an English doctor, published a book entitled "Western Diseases and Their Emergence and Prevention." In it he discusses the findings of some incredible research that he conducted. He compared the diets of rural Africans and the British naval officers stationed near them. The Africans had diets consisting mainly of high fiber fruits and vegetables and the naval officers had diets consisting mainly of meat, refined white flour, and sugar. The Africans had normal bowel movements eighteen to thirty-six hours after eating and the naval officers had difficult bowel movements seventy-two to one hundred hours after eating. The naval officers also developed a number of conditions including colorectal cancers, coronary artery disease, high blood pressure, diabetes, obesity, high cholesterol, diverticulitis and hemorrhoids. The Africans did not have a significant presence of any of these conditions until they switched to the British diet.

The human body needs over fifty different nutrients to feed it and to produce healthy, new cells. The quality of those cells depends upon the nutrients available in the body. If you are not giving your body what it needs to create healthy new cells, the cells will be "defective," fewer in number and more easily damaged or destroyed.

The immune system is the doctor that lives within the human body. It is designed to be on duty at all times, vigilantly protecting our bodies from foreign invaders, including defective cells. If you are following habits that reduce the effectiveness of your immune system, you are vulnerable to attack.

Taken together, the production of weakened, defective cells and a weakened immune system create the perfect storm for sickness and disease in humans. Science has ignored this perfect storm for whatever reason, so it doesn't yet have a name. I call it the Cumulative Effect.

The Cumulative Effect
We look at other species nearing extinction with fleeting pangs of guilt. We think, "Oh how terrible that we are destroying the habitat of that poor salamander. There will be no more on this planet some day soon. All progress is not good progress," we think. "Poor salamanders… Never had a chance against those bulldozers…Mmm… I wonder if Sports Center is on yet."

We are destroying the habitat and/or polluting the ecosystem of countless species and, ultimately, see it as an inevitable consequence of the progress of mankind. Unfortunately, what we can't seem to see quite as well is that we are doing the same thing to our own species. We are destroying and polluting our natural habitat and the first sign of the weakening of our species is setting in – an epidemic of incurable disease. By changing the environment in which we live, I believe that we have retriggered natural selection on our species (and others) and the epidemic of degenerative diseases is one of the end results.

Think I'm crazy? Consider this: the environment in which our bodies operate today is remarkably different than that of our grandparents, great-grandparents, great, and great-grandparents and every generation that has come before us. How different? In modern countries, more chemical toxins (pesticides, herbicides, antibiotics, chlorine, lead, pharmaceutical drugs, etc.) enter our bodies in one month than *ever* entered our great grandparents' bodies! And, because we have become increasingly sedentary and changed our diets so significantly in the past five decades, our bodies cannot dispose of those toxins at the rate at which they enter. Dr. Don Colbert, a noted physician and author wrote, "A chronic, low-dose accumulation of toxic matter eventually puts stress on the immune system and may pollute the blood stream and every cell and organ in the body." So, we have a toxic buildup in the body (what some refer to as the body's toxic load) that our ancestors never had. And to compound things, our immune systems are suppressed in a way they have never been before as a result of the combination of accumulating toxins and poor lifestyle habits (like an increased consumption of simple sugar, which impairs immune function).

Unfortunately, this is not the only significant difference between the environment in which our bodies operate and the environment in which our ancestors' bodies operated. Most of the food we eat today is processed, and has very little nutrition in comparison to the food our ancestors ate. And we tend to eat more calories and lead more sedentary lives than our ancestors. The impact these lifestyle changes have on healthy cell reproduction should not be underestimated.

Think about what would happen if terrorists that were committed to causing harm in any way possible were streaming into the United States or Great Britain at a time when the countries had let their national defense and intelligence systems dwindle. The terrorists would roam free, setting up networks and working together. They would be able to act in completely unpredictable ways and the countries would not be able to protect themselves. The terrorists would attack again and again unchecked, weakening infrastructure and causing chaos and ruin.

This is exactly what is going on at a cellular and molecular level in the human body to cause such an epidemic of sickness in the modern world. Foreign invaders are streaming into the body and attacking molecules, genes, cells and tissues and our defenses are weakened so there is no means to effectively stop the attack. At the same time, the body is reproducing ever-weaker cells in ever-weaker organs and systems throughout the body. Eventually, the body becomes so weak and damaged that sickness and disease form. *This* is the central cause for the epidemic described at the beginning of this book. *This* is what I call the Cumulative Effect.

The Cumulative Effect is the phrase I use to describe what is going on in our bodies that, I believe, is the central cause of the epidemic of the chronic illness and degenerative disease facing the modern world today. As illustrated in the picture below, there are far more toxins entering the body than are leaving it, resulting in an accumulation of a deadly witch's brew. The body's immune system, weakened by poor habits, is unable to effectively fight off the accumulating toxins, allowing chemical and biological reactions to occur unchecked and leaving the body vulnerable to genetic and molecular damage. At the same time, the body's regenerative functions are impaired, impacting cells, tissue and, ultimately, entire systems in the body. The combined effect, a perfect storm so-to-speak, degenerates the body, leaving it open to chronic disease, the flavor of the disease determined by the specific damage and toxins accumulating in the body and your genetic predisposition.

The Cumulative Effect

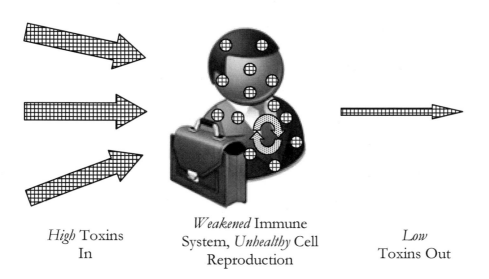

High Toxins
In

Weakened Immune
System, *Unhealthy* Cell
Reproduction

Low
Toxins Out

I believe that most of the chronic illnesses and degenerative diseases that afflict Western society today are a direct result of the Cumulative Effect – an accumulation of toxins in the body along with a weakened immune system and unhealthy cell reproduction. This epidemic is not the result of hereditary bad luck or chance encounters with rare, lethal substances. It is not the result of a few bad men at a fireworks factory in Toledo, Ohio, or a religious curse brought on by Muslim hatred of the West. It is a self-inflicted, life-threatening wound.

This is only my hypothesis. I just made the point that our science is not mature enough to prove this beyond all reasonable doubt. And we have the option of waiting (and waiting) on our science to mature enough to fully test this hypothesis in a double-blind, placebo controlled environment. But do we really need to wait what could be hundreds of years when we can *already* perfectly correlate the meteoric rise in chronic illness and degenerative disease to the dramatic increase in the use of synthetic chemicals, the widespread practice of industrial agriculture, the increase of processed food in the modern diet and the adoption of poor lifestyle habits in Western culture? Do we need the Surgeon General to hold a news conference and issue a formal warning when we can already link hundreds of chemicals directly to human health problems? Do we need a big brand company to tell us that "four out of five doctors" agree that bad lifestyle habits result in an impaired immune system and weakened cell and tissue development?

Think this through for a minute. Do we?

We're humans. We rule the earth. Science and profit are sets of rules we made up ourselves. They don't control us – we control them. Certainly we can change the rules if the survival of our species is at risk, right?

And this isn't an *impeding* crisis, either. This isn't some grandfather's this-country-is-going-to-hell-in-a-hand-basket concern with a shred of truth that you put in the back of your mind to pull out later when it's time to get serious about it. This thing is now.

Although the environmental crisis and the energy crisis are serious and require our attention, the reality is that their impact is ahead of us. The disease epidemic isn't. It is hitting us now. When you look around at the rate of degenerative disease, you can only conclude that the crisis is upon us already. It has overcome us like a wave while we weren't paying attention. All of a sudden you look up and one-fifth of the people you know have some kind of chronic health problem and maybe one out of every eight to ten people you know has some form of degenerative disease. I don't care what some doctor or special interest statistician says – that's not normal. That is not how our species has lived up to now.

In the recent remake of the movie *The War of the Worlds,* aliens invade earth and their superior weapons quickly overpower the defenses of our military. The aliens roam the earth killing hundreds of thousands of people without any significant resistance. The world dissolves into chaos as panic-stricken people run in every direction looking for cover. Then, when it seems that the aliens have achieved dominion over the earth, they begin to falter. They stray from their mission, act erratically and, without explanation, begin to die. Human life on earth is spared, but not because of the heroics of a Hollywood muscleman. We learn at the conclusion of the movie that the aliens got sick from the germs, viruses and infections that they encountered on earth. The immune systems of the humans, the movie narrator tells the audience, had developed resistance against these common earthly ailments. The invaders, however, had never encountered such "alien" threats, and their immune systems were unable to defend them against them.

It struck me as I reflected on the unexpected conclusion of this science fiction flick that we humans are going through something very similar. Our immune systems are prepared to fight against earthly bacterial infections, viruses and germs because humans have been dealing with them since the beginning of time. However, our immune systems, in their weakened state, are suddenly encountering hundreds of alien substances – synthetic chemicals, genetically modified food, chemically altered food, etc. – introduced within the last three to four decades, and we, not unlike the aliens in *The War of the Worlds,* are beginning to falter.

Anything that creates a sudden shift in the delicate harmony that took thousands of years to create is deadly to those that coexisted in that harmony. I am not a doom and gloom kind of guy, but, unfortunately, it is improbable that our species can adapt fast enough to the change that has happened and is continuing to happen in the world in which we exist. Because of the pace of change and the slow speed of animal adaptation, we will continue to move further and further out of harmony with our environment. It is also highly unlikely that we can shift our environment back to the way it was – the way our bodies expect it to be.
So, if we cannot adapt fast enough to our changing surroundings and we can't turn our surroundings back to the way they were, what's left? If the Cumulative Effect is, indeed, the cause of the epidemic of chronic illness that is already upon the modern world, we will have to deal with it. Naturally, we have to identify it, diagnose it and cure it. But

unfortunately, because of the nature of the Cumulative Effect, we won't be able to develop a *cure* in the near future, at least in the traditional sense of the word "cure."

When you and I think of a "cure," we typically imagine a vaccine. Most of us believe that some day there will be an immunization against cancer like there is for rubella. Thoughts of a cure might conjure up images of booster shots given to children that prevent diseases like cancer. Unfortunately, this is a fantasy. There cannot be a vaccine against degenerative diseases caused by The Cumulative Effect in any of our lifetimes. The number and complexity of the chemical reactions going on at a molecular level inside our bodies far exceeds our science. Since the chronic illnesses that would result from the Cumulative Effect are caused by a myriad of complex interactions in the body that exceed our understanding today, there could not be a singular cure for them. And as for the poor lifestyle habits that are weakening our immune defenses, well, there just ain't a pill for that!

While there can be no cure for the diseases resulting from the Cumulative Effect in our lifetime, fortunately, as you will read in the upcoming chapter, it is possible to *prevent* the Cumulative Effect from occurring. I have found that we can, to a large extent, control our personal environment, our bubble, so to speak, by changing our individual habits so that we mostly encounter our environment in a way that our bodies expect. By following routines that reduce our exposure to synthetic toxins, increase the elimination of those toxins that do get into our bodies, and improve immune health, we can *prevent the cause* of most chronic illness and degenerative disease from occurring in our bodies.

Chapter 4

Health 102: Habits Determine Health

Nothing is stronger than habit.
Ovid

I remember it vividly. It was the seventh grade. We all knew it was coming. The older kids had told us about it on the bus. Over the course of two weeks in health class, we sat in our seats fighting off the giggles as the teacher held up plastic genitals naming their parts and describing their functions. It was fantastic to hear a teacher say those words. I mean, seriously, it was wildly funny to hear your seventh grade teacher say "vulva," "scrotum," "labia," and "pubic" in front of your class. These were outstanding words for a 7th grader to hear an adult say. And, of course, we promptly told the sixth graders on the bus all about it.

Unfortunately, our teacher was telling us about something we already knew about in the seventh grade (I am embarrassed to admit). It was still memorable, but mostly because Mrs. Pierce held a plastic wiener in her hand the whole time she talked to us one day. To be sure, all of us that sat through her class have successfully practiced what she talked about by now – a lot. However, as I sat thinking about Health 101 while writing this book, reproductive anatomy is all I really remember. I remember a great deal about math and science, English and social studies. I even remember a lot about art, woodshop and home economics. But I couldn't tell you what we learned in health, other than words like *semen* and *urethra*.

We go to school for an average of 13 years in the West and we learn a lot about a lot of subjects: geometry, poetry, government, algebra, literature, science, foreign language, art, computers, history, drama, politics, and more. Yet we get a few hours of basic instruction on how to pilot this incredibly complex organism called the human body in which we live for an average of nearly 80 years – and the most memorable part of the instruction is how to use your genitals for pleasure. Does that seem right? Shouldn't operating the only body we will ever get be the one thing we learn the most about?

Was there a separation of health and state at some point? Why don't we teach our young people how to keep themselves vigorously healthy? Shouldn't we spend as much time learning about nutrition as we do about nouns? Does it make sense that we learn more about the oboe than we learn about obesity? Why would we learn more in school about sculpture than we do about stress?

In America, most people live with the belief that they are the healthiest nation in the world. In the 2007 Preventative Health Survey, when asked how healthy they considered themselves to be, participants overwhelmingly responded that they were either in average or above average health.

How healthy do you consider yourself to be?

Answer	0%	100%	Response Ratio
Healthier than the average person			45%
In average health			48%
Less healthy than the average person			6%
No Response(s)			<1%

It is not surprising, then, that we learn as much about hexagons as we do about human health in school. Americans have a general feeling of health and well being. They believe that they are just fine, thanks.

While Americans do have a high standard of living, a low rate of infectious and contagious disease, and access to the most advanced emergency medical treatment and general health-care in the world, we are actually among the developed world's least healthy people. Americans are facing epidemic proportions of degenerative diseases like cancer, cardiovascular disease, hypertension, arthritis, dementia and osteoporosis.

How could this be? How could the wealthiest nation on earth be home to one of the world's most advanced academic systems, possess the most advanced technologies and house the world's leading medical companies and still be among the world's most unhealthy people? It is a complex answer, but one that has a lot to do with the fact that Americans never really learn how to operate the complex body they're born with. Our learning about human health comes, instead, from special interests –

those who really only have a *special interest* in how much money we spend with them.

Although it may be all we remember from health class, health is not the act of intercourse or the resulting reproduction. Health is not big muscles, ripped abs and shiny white teeth like you see in the movies. Health is not a kelp milkshake, a tree bark energy bar and a handful of exotic herbs like you hear from the clerk in the health food store. Health is not a secret the government doesn't want you to know about and it's not an energy force you can tune into like you might read in popular books.

Very simply, health is a sustained state where we are free from sickness of any kind. Healthy people are those who have an absence of sickness and the ability to maintain that state. Healthy people, as you will see below, derive their health – their freedom from sickness of any kind – from their daily choices, or more specifically, their habits.

Habits Determine Health

Michael Leavitt, health and human services secretary under George W. Bush, was being interviewed for a January 2006 article in *Newsweek* magazine and was asked by the interviewer, "What do you think is the biggest thing that could improve America's health?" Mr. Leavitt replied, "Focusing on wellness instead of treatment. We're seeing an epidemic of chronic disease. Obesity is one example. And we can improve by changing our habits and focusing on our health."

Habit is defined in Webster's dictionary as "an acquired behavior pattern regularly followed until it has become almost involuntary." Said even more simply, a habit is a routine that you regularly follow without thought or special effort. You just do it.

When I get into my car, I buckle my seatbelt. I always have. I don't have to be reminded to do it. It happens automatically as if done by a machine. As soon as my rear end hits the car seat and my feet are in front of the pedals, my right hand automatically reaches across my body, grabs the metal tab, pulls it to the right and inserts it into the buckle. It is a habit and I do it without thinking.

I have found that habits, these involuntary routines, actually determine a lot about life for all living creatures. I have a large wooded area behind my home and am fortunate to get to see and experience a lot of wildlife from my kitchen window every day. Deer are quite abundant in these woods and my family and I enjoy watching them, especially in the fall and winter when the leaves are off the trees. We began to notice that we would see the same deer in the same places at the same times every day. You could almost set your watch by them. They are so consistent that there are well worn paths traversing the edge of the woods where they walk every day. These deer, like me with my seatbelt, have habits that they follow automatically every day, rain or shine, summer or winter.

It turns out that habits determine a lot about life as we know it including our health. The routines that we follow on a daily basis, usually without much thought, are the primary determinants of our health. I'll say this again because it is the single most important statement in this book: *the habits that you have formed in your life, the things that you do automatically, every day without any forethought, by and large determine your health.* They determine whether you will get a disease, how you will spend your senior years, and how and when you will die.

Please read that statement again. If after reading it and rereading it, you don't know this to be the truth, if your subconscious is not screaming at you that this is the truth about health, if you do not have the feeling that this affirms what your gut has been telling you all along – that all these quick fixes and health gimmicks peddled in the media were too good to be true – then put down this book. You are not ready to go on. You cannot possibly benefit from what the remainder of this book can tell you.

But if you have been nodding your head in agreement as you read these pages, if you know in your very bones that health is complex to screw up and, therefore, not mended with quick fixes and silver bullets, if you feel that there is real truth in the notion that habits are the foundation of health – read on. This is the best investment of time that you could possibly make. After all, your health is your single greatest asset.

There are three basic reasons that habits determine health:

Reason #1: You Are the Sum of Your Habits. The average person living in America today lives for 28,324 days. In that time span, a person eats over 100,000 meals and snacks, drinks over 100,000 servings of beverages and uses synthetic products in his house or on his body at least

80,000 times. He encounters at least 50,000 sources of stress and anxiety, has 28,324 opportunities for restful sleep and has at least 20,000 opportunities to be active. In his life, the average American has nearly 3,000 opportunities to shop for groceries or influence the grocery shopping and visits a restaurant at least that many times.

These activities number in the hundreds of thousands and they all affect human health in some way. Taken individually, each activity does not have a major impact on health. However, when taken as a whole over the course of 10, 15 or 20 years, they have a significant affect on health – either positive or negative.

Most people don't really acknowledge how many unhealthy actions they take on a daily basis. Unfortunately, health is very poorly understood by most people. Often, people think that the unhealthy person is that obese uncle that smokes, drinks alcohol to excess, eats pepperoni pizza four nights per week and sleeps an average of five hours per night. He probably is very unhealthy but, very likely, so is the sedentary woman who eats margarine on her bagel, has a stressful life and constantly drinks diet cola with artificial sweetener.

Over time, if unhealthy actions persist, health is compromised and chronic illness can develop. Let me be clearer: outside of a freak exposure to large quantities of radiation or other harmful toxins, you couldn't spontaneously cause degenerative disease or chronic illness if you tried. It is impossible to suddenly bring on arthritis, cancer, Alzheimer's, cardiovascular disease, hypertension, dementia, lupus, osteoporosis or any other degenerative disease. You have to work at it. It takes years and years of poor choices banging away at your well-fortified health like the cannons of an enemy garrison. Eventually, after a sustained barrage of attacks on your health, the array of unhealthy choices becomes too much for the body to fight off, and it gives in. The body's natural defenses break down and its systems are besieged by the toxins that are a consequence of the harmful choices that we make. The toxins degrade the cells and tissues of the body (in ways that we don't yet fully understand) and the body lacks the nutrition to reproduce healthy cells, which creates effects such as mutations of DNA, the degradation of the body's systems, or the stimulation of the immune system to attack the body itself, leading eventually to what we know as chronic disease.

Interesting, but not earth-shattering, right? Well, here's the point: nearly all of the actions that we take are the result of our habits. Nearly all of the hundreds of thousands of choices that we make that affect our health, positively or negatively, are a result of routines that we follow automatically without thought. The foods you eat, how much food you eat, the amount of sleep you get, your restaurant choices, the foods you select at those restaurant, how you react to stress, the beverages you choose, how many beverages you drink, when and how often you are physically active, the products you choose at the grocery store, and the synthetic products you use on your body and in your home – all of it is largely habitual.

As much as 85% of the actions that affect health are a result of your daily habits. Random events make up only 10% - 15% of the actions in your life. The summary of your actions over time is heavily weighted to your habits.

You may feel as though you are not a creature of habit, but ask yourself the following questions about the last 60 days:

- How many times did you go to sleep and wake up at times dramatically different from the norm for you?
- What percent of the food you bought at the grocery store was something new and different for you?
- How many times did you try something you don't normally order when you went to a restaurant?
- How many new/ different beverages (type not brand) did you try?
- How many fruits or vegetables did you try that you do not routinely eat?
- Did your physical activity regimen vary greatly from the norm?
- Did you change more than one or two of the synthetic products that you typically use (shampoo, soap, toothpaste, shaving cream, mouthwash, lotion, detergent, dish soap, glass cleaner, toilet cleaner, wood polish, fertilizer, weed killer, pest control, etc.)?

The behaviors that we follow, the actions that we take, very often unconsciously and out of habit, are the things that determine our health. Your daily routines determine the toxins that enter and leave your body, the overall wellbeing of your immune system, and your body's ability to reproduce healthy cells. Your health and, to a great degree, your longevity depend upon the habits that you have most likely settled into, not chosen, in your life.

Reason #2: Habits are Automatic. Habits are performed involuntarily. The mind and body perform habits routinely, without thinking. And because the body craves the physical, mental and/or emotional stimulus it gets from its habits, there is a dependence on habits that supports their continuation.

Traditionally, being healthy has meant having to think: eat this, avoid that, don't include this, and do include that. It can be cumbersome to plan. How can a person possibly remember to accomplish all of the health recommendations made by the media – eat coleslaw, blueberries, almonds, green tea, red wine, dark chocolate, broccoli; avoid margarine, trans fats, MSG, corn syrup, processed food, NutraSweet, saccharine; get plenty of exercise, sleep and clean water; and reduce your weight and stress…?

If it is not already a habit, remembering to do something that is good for us requires constant effort. In order for us to consistently repeat a healthy behavior that is not a habit, we must vigilantly think about doing it over and over and over again. Typically, we fail because of the discipline and effort that is required to keep up that behavior day after day. Just think about how many of your "eat healthy - lose weight - exercise more" resolutions have failed. Our habits end up winning. They dominate our behavior because they happen automatically.

This is because *habits result in repeated behaviors without consistent effort.* Regardless of our motivation or good intentions, our attention span is too short to effect meaningful change by willpower alone. Habits allow you to take the planning and thinking out of being healthy. For example, I eat fruit and whole grain cereal for breakfast every day and I focus on eating primarily vegetables for dinner. I always drink water while I work out and as I am going to bed at night. These are habits for me and I rarely deviate from them. I don't have to think about them or plan for them. They aren't even choices anymore. They just happen.

My body craves these behaviors because I have been doing them long enough that it expects them. The simplest example is the seatbelt. For those of you who wear your seatbelt habitually, what happens when you don't have a seatbelt on? You feel naked, like you are unsafely flying through space, right? You feel like something is missing, like something isn't right. That is because your body is craving the stimulus, the restraint and pressure across your chest and shoulders, that it feels when it senses the motion of the car.

Habits work because they result in behavior change far more easily than consciously changing your actions. The body has a natural "infrastructure" that supports the repetition of behaviors and it can be leveraged for health. Consider the following differences between *changes of action* and *habits*:

> *Change of Action*: I need to eat more fruits, vegetables and grains.
> *Habit*: I will only eat whole grain cereal with fruit for breakfast and a vegetable plate or salad for lunch.

> *Change of Action*: I need to drink more water and less coffee and soda.
> *Habit*: I will drink one bottle of water during my workout, one bottle of water on the commute to work, one bottle on the commute home and one bottle in bed while reading.

> *Change of Action*: I need to get more sleep.
> *Habit*: I will get in bed by 9:00 p.m., read for one hour, go to sleep by 10:00 p.m., and wake up every day at 6:00 a.m.

Do you see the difference? Can you see how a change of action requires consistent thought and effort and a habit can simply happen? Can you imagine how much easier it would be to improve your health by changing your habits?

Reason #3: Habits are Hard to Break. As a young person, you adopt the habits that your parents have, particularly as it relates to food. You eat what your parents buy and serve. You become accustomed to the tastes, textures, smells and appearance of the food served in your home day in and day out. When you first venture out of the home to eat on your own (at school, for example) you favor the foods served at home. You trust that food and you know what to expect. The same familial pattern holds true for physical activity, rest, how you handle stress, how you manage your weight, and the overall responsibility you take for your health.

This tends to follow you through your youth, but once a person forms a stable home of his or her own and, in particular, once he or she marries, a whole new set of environmental factors influence the formation of new habits. Although you retain many of the habits that you grew up around, you also tend to adopt some of the habits that your spouse and her family follow and even form entirely new habits based on friendships, work and cultural surroundings.

Although your environment has much to do with what habits you will adopt, your own body helps to reinforce them so that they become routine. It turns out that the human brain and body prefer a rhythm, a ritual. For example, as you begin to get into a regular work schedule as a young adult, your body begins to settle into a pattern. You get tired at the same time each night and tend to wake up at roughly the same time in the morning, even when your alarm does not go off. You tend to get hungry at the same times every day, depending on what and when you are accustomed to eating. You even tend to have bowel movements at the same time, probably also depending on when you eat (and sleep). The same is true for every mental and/or physical routine that you follow. You get into a program and the body adjusts itself to that program and tends to resist change.

Unless your life is utter chaos, your body has a rhythm to which it is biologically, chemically and neurologically adjusted. The body's systems have become adjusted, some say almost dependent, on the stimulus that your typical patterns provide. The body prefers the routines, regimens and rhythms to which it has become accustomed – like sleep. Have you ever noticed how bad you feel when you change your sleeping pattern – going to bed later or getting up earlier - for just a few days? Your body expects to be on the routine to which you have trained it and it loses its way when it does not receive the "inputs" that it is expecting.

I do a lot of domestic and international travel. As a result, I often travel to other time zones and, while my routine stays largely the same, the hours shift because of the time difference. When this happens, my body resists the change. It wants to go to sleep, wake up, eat, exercise and do everything else on its standard schedule. After several days of resisting, the body begins to adjust gradually to the new time zone, but I still don't feel quite right. But when I come home, I seem to snap right back into my regular schedule almost immediately and I feel great. It is as if my body is thanking me for getting it back into its comfortable old routine.

Because our bodies are complex and resilient, they only change over time and, as a result, the human body adapts slowly. Like a large oil tanker at sea that takes time to turn, our bodies prefer the course on which they are sailing. To successfully change its rhythms, the body has to be re-trained gradually and methodically. If you try to change too fast, you don't have the biological, chemical and neurological support and your brain and body will pull you back into the pattern that it is expecting you to follow.

I hope you can see how habits determine health. This is because: 1) we are the sum of our habits, 2) habits happen automatically, and 3) habits are hard to break. Except in rare circumstances like a chemical contamination, our health is not destroyed in an instant. It is slowly and continually degraded until the body is so damaged that diseases begin to set in. As cold and harsh as it sounds, the truth is that most degenerative disease is self-inflicted. Occasionally, it the result of abusive indulgences like alcoholism, but far more often, it is the result of a life of poor habits formed unconsciously out of convenience, human nature, taste and marketing. It is easy to see, then, why the habits that we follow day in and day out for years are what determine our health.

Making Habits Work for You
Have you ever started a new exercise program and failed to keep up the new habit? Have you tried to lose weight or eat healthier and been unable to make it stick? It is probably because you did not have the support system that your brain and body needed to get "re-programmed."

As discussed earlier, the brain and body become accustomed, even dependent, upon the routines that you follow. When you try to change, the brain and body, expecting the stimulus provided by the customary routines, literally crave the expected stimulus. You sense the cravings – a candy bar after lunch, a cigarette during the commute, an evening on the couch instead of in the gym – and you probably fight them for a while. However, we all have moments of weakness, and we give in to the cravings. One moment of weakness justifies another and another, and pretty soon, you brain and body have pulled you back into the old routine.

Making sudden changes in lifestyle is difficult because of the principle of inertia. Things in motion tend to stay in motion. Our impatient, instant-gratification way of life leads us to think that sudden change is necessary, and our pride and stubbornness leads us to believe that it is possible. Adopting new habits or breaking old ones is nearly *im*possible to do using the cold turkey approach.

However, things in motion can change direction little by little. The key to changing habits, it turns out, is subtleness, not suddenness. To change one's habits, one needs to be clever, not bold. The body must be re-trained to expect a new habit and this isn't achieved with resolve and force of will alone.

Breaking and forming habits is not hard, as we've come to believe. It is actually quite simple – it just requires a smarter approach.

I am an industrial engineer by education with a specific focus on human behavior. For over a decade, my colleagues and I have worked with some of the largest companies in the world to help them change the *habits* of their employees in a company that I co-created called Knowlagent. These companies hired us to more closely align the behavior of their frontline employees with their corporate objectives. The theory went that, if you could get the average and poor-performing frontline employees to more consistently act like the top performers in the company, the company could sell a lot more stuff and more effectively retain customers. The frontline employees were the ones interacting with the customers and, if they consistently followed the habits that had proven success for the best performers, their results would improve.

Over the years of working with hundreds of thousands of people, we found that, in order for people to successfully change one or more habits, they had to take advantage of the inertia of their existing habits and then continuously apply subtle changes for a period of time. To create this environment of habit formation, we found that people needed a progressive routine repeated over time. Said another way, we found the four ingredients of habit-building were *progression*, *routines*, *repetition* and *time*.

- **Progression** – New habits are not formed all at once. Habit change is about subtleness, not suddenness. A ship at sail changes course slowly. Behavior change happens in much the same way.

- **Routines** – In order to adopt a habit, a person must have a structure in place that reminds him to follow certain behaviors. Without that structure, even with the best intentions, we tend to give in to our brain/body cravings for the stimulus it expects or to follow the path of least resistance. The most reliable support structure for permanently changing lifestyle habits is the daily routine.

- **Repetition** – Repetition is important in changing habits. The brain and body need to regularly practice the new habit in order for it to become an expected stimulus. Frequency makes a path a trail.

- **Time** – I bet you have heard the old adage, '21 days to make a habit.' It turns out that the time that it takes to make a habit depends upon several environmental factors that differ by person and habit. Generally, in 20 to 30 days, a consistently repeated behavior becomes habitual because your mind and body adjusts to it. It becomes the path of least resistance.

New Habit = Progression + Routines + Repetition + Time

The problem most people have when they try change their habits is that they try to do it all at once. They rely on willpower to try and overcome a routine and don't realize that they have to also overcome mental and physical "cravings" for their old habits. In order to be successful at changing your habits, you must progressively develop a new habit leveraging an existing one that already has momentum (that your body is expecting). In addition, a new routine has to be formed to support the changed habit so that old routines that helped to form the old habit don't pull you back in. And, most importantly, you have to repeat the changed habit for long enough that your body begins to expect the new stimulus. Most people don't have all of those elements when they set out to change their actions and, as a result, they often fail.

To effectively form a new habit, you need **P**rogression, **R**outines, **R**epetition and **T**ime. Not surprisingly, my approach to habit adoption is called PRRT (pronounced "pert" – creative genius runs in my family). PRRT is a simple, proven approach for adopting new habits that leverages the functioning of the human body. PRRT takes advantage of the inertia of your existing habits and uses subtle changes, daily routines and repetition to change habits over time.

In Part III of this book, I included my PRRT system for changing your habits. My system is extremely easy to understand and apply to your life. It is practical and realistic for people of all ages. But for now, just internalize this: *The key to getting well and staying well is very simple – change your habits.*

The Habits of Healthy People
Did you ever have a pet fish? Imagine with me a pet goldfish living in a small one-gallon fish bowl. This fish bowl has blue rocks on the bottom, a plastic plant and a ceramic sunken ship sitting on the rocks. Day in and day out, every day, this is where the fish lives. This is the fish's "individual environment."

Now imagine that a toxic chemical in the cheap paint on the blue rocks begins to seep unnoticeably into the water in that fishbowl. Regardless of how many times the water is changed, the rocks in that fishbowl pollute the fish's environment. Also imagine that the fish's owner begins to feed the fish a synthetic fish food that the fish was never meant to eat. Now the fish lives in this unhealthy environment and he is eating food that is not healthy for his body, day in and day out, every day. Eventually, you can imagine that the fish will become sick, get some kind of chronic fishy sickness, and wind up a floater. His individual environment is unhealthy and cannot sustain him. Poor fishy.

Habits are to humans what a fishbowl is to a fish. Our daily routines pretty well define who we are and how we live. Habits form a human's "individual environment." If you have habits that are unhealthy; your individual environment is unhealthy just like the fish's. Like the fish, if you live in an unhealthy individual environment over time, you will probably get some kind of chronic illness and you might even wind up a floater before your time. Poor human.

But unlike the poor fish stuck in the toxic fishbowl eating whatever its owner feeds it, humans *can* adopt healthy habits and move from an unhealthy "fishbowl" to a healthy one. By changing our habits, we create a *new* individual environment for ourselves. Changing our habits can put our bodies back into harmony with nature, reduce the Cumulative Effect on us, improve our immune systems and improve the health of our bodies' life-sustaining systems, enabling us to live longer, more vigorous lives.

Earlier, I described the Cumulative Effect. I described how our synthetic environment puts us into contact with dozens of toxic chemicals every day, many of which enter our bodies and never leave. I also described how the unhealthy habits of the modern man or woman reduced the effectiveness of the body's natural healing system and impaired the body's life-sustaining, regenerative functions. The combination of these things – toxins entering the body and staying there, a weakened immune system and impaired regenerative functions – results in a condition called The Cumulative Effect, which I have come to believe is the source of most of the chronic illness and degenerative disease in the world today.

Below, in contrast to the illustration of The Cumulative Effect included in an earlier chapter, is an illustration of what I believe happens when someone adopts and follows The 8 Habits of Healthy People.

Healthy People Follow Habits That Beat the Cumulative Effect

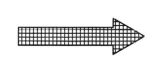 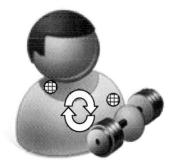 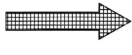

| *Reduced* Toxins In | *Strong* Immune System, *Healthy* Cell Reproduction | *Increased* Toxins Out |

In this picture, our cartoon man has fewer toxins accumulating in his body because his habits reduce the amount of synthetic toxins he comes into contact with and help to increase the flow of toxins leaving the body. In addition, his habits support his body's immune system and its life-sustaining functions, enabling them to effectively protect and sustain healthy genes, cells and tissue. In effect, this picture illustrates health. It illustrates the condition that modern man should strive to achieve in order to live a long healthy life.

Following habits of health enables a person to create an "individual environment" that is healthier than the modern world.

When it comes to fighting sickness and disease, following healthy habits reduces toxins entering your body, increases the number of toxins that you eliminate from your body, enhances the body's ability to reproduce healthy cells, and improves the functioning of the body's immune system. All of these benefits improve overall health. However, there is one benefit that is more important than all of the rest.

The Doctor Within
Within you, there is a doctor that is always on call. He works 24 hours a day, seven days a week, including holidays. He never takes a vacation. He has no other patients and works only for you. He doesn't charge you any money, he is extremely convenient, and there is no waiting. There is no paperwork, no weigh in, no cups to pee in, no blood to draw, no tongue depressors and no co-pay. Most importantly, he knows everything there is to know about your complex chemistry, biology and molecular structure and has remedies for thousands of germs, viruses, bacteria, infections and problems that occur in your body.

Who is this incredible doctor?

It is your immune system, or what I like to call *the doctor within*.

The human body is a complex and resilient organism with its own healing system. This sophisticated system protects the body against the thousands of attacks made upon it daily by bacteria, microorganisms, toxins, etc. It can diagnose illness or injury, seek it out wherever it may have spread in the body, and heal itself. It has even been able to adapt somewhat as man has developed through the years and become able to fortify us against everything but the most acute and severe attacks.

It is really amazing to think about the wide range of things that can happen to our bodies – thousands of different bacteria, viruses, fungi, venomous bug bites, and hundreds of potential broken bones, lacerations, abrasions, etc. Our immune system must be capable of dealing with all of these things at a moments notice. At this very moment, your immune system is working hard to fight off thousands of foreign invaders inside your body.

In fact, most illnesses and injury that we encounter (stomach upset, back pain, pink eye, ear infection, etc.) end by themselves as a result of our healing system going to work. Just like when you cut your finger and the body heals itself on the outside, the immune system operates under the surface repairing itself at the molecular and cellular level. If you are sick or in pain or dealing with bumps, bites or a rash; if you've got a cut or scrape, an infection or a cold, your immune system is fighting as hard as it possibly can, nonstop, without rest, to get you well.

Your immune system includes your lymphatic system, a network of vessels and lymph nodes that transports and filters lymph fluid, the appendix, the tonsils, the adenoids, gut-associated lymphoid tissue and bone marrow. This sophisticated system enables the body to distinguish "self" from "non-self" and is capable of launching an attack on what it considers non-self using the body's most effective weapon, the antibody. Foreign invaders like viruses, bacteria, insect venoms, mutated cells, pollen and chemicals are known as antigens. When an antigen shows up in the body and comes into contact with cells from the immune system, protein molecules called antibodies are produced specifically to fight the type of antigen that has been identified. Those antibodies are designed by the immune system to seek out and destroy only the antigens. Typically, when the body encounters an antigen that it has not encountered before, the production of antibodies takes about one week. However, once the immune system has dealt with a specific antigen, say a type of virus, it can produce antibodies much more rapidly in the future.

Your body's healing system is far superior to anything that man can conceive of or manufacture. It has all of the answers and most of the cures. It can respond with a lethal attack, specifically designed for what ails you (with no unintended consequences or "side effects"). And, if you take care of it, it will not only heal you when you get sick, but it will prevent you from getting sick in the first place. For these reasons and many more, your immune system, the doctor within you, should be relied upon as your primary protection against sickness and disease.

Why Do You Think They Call It Immune?
The healthier (and more health-obsessed) I become, the more I pay attention to the health of the people around me. Over the last few years while writing this book, I have made a conscious effort to observe the general health of the people in my life. I pay attention to their habits and I pay attention to their ailments.

This empirical study of the people in my life has confirmed a few things about health in my mind. First, generally speaking, there is a group of people (about 1 in 10) in my life that rarely get sick (colds, flu, etc.). Then, there is a group of people (about 5 in 10) that get sick two to three times per year. Finally, there is a group of people (about 4 in 10) that get sick far more often, typically five to six times per year.

This last group, the group of people that is sick more often than the others, is really interesting to me because I used to be one of them. I notice that this chronic cold and flu bunch doesn't just get sick often, they get *really* sick, often. They go down for the count. Also, the frequently sick have illnesses that tend to stay with them longer than the people who are sick less frequently. Their symptoms linger and they vacilate for weeks between getting better and getting worse.

This empirical analysis of the few hundred people in my life is significant because it demonstrates something very important to me. As you might expect to see when dealing with a group of associated (not random) people, the people in my not-so-scientific study are nearly all from the same demographic. They are all from roughly the same socioeconomic group and geographic area. Heck, most of the few hundred people in my life work together, sharing the same air and working conditions five days per week. Yet, despite the homogeneity, despite the sameness in their lives, they have differences in their incidence of sickness. One group rarely gets colds and flu, one group gets colds and flu two to three times per year, and one group gets colds and flu five or more times per year.

Why? These people encounter the same bacteria and viruses in their daily lives, in general. What causes this difference? If their environment is generally the same, there must be something different about the people.

Very simply, it is the health of their immune system (which is a function of their habits). The immune system's primary job is to keep a person healthy despite all of the forces that are pushing him in the direction of illness. It is the human body's defense in the war against sickness and disease. If you get sick a lot, in means that your body's defense is not able to effectively fight off foreign attackers and illness. If you do not get sick very often, it generally means that your immune system is doing a good job of responding to, and destroying, foreign invaders. In other words, the frequency, severity and duration of the colds and flu that one gets are a perfect measure of the health of one's immune system. If you get sick a lot, get *very* sick from time to time, and/or have symptoms of sickness that hang around for weeks, you probably have a weakened immune system due to unhealthy habits.

That might be okay if the consequences of a weakened immune system were simply a gravely voice and the sniffles, but because your immune system is the critical element in your fight against *all* foreign invaders in your body, a weakened immune system makes you vulnerable to chronic illness and disease. Remember, I said above that the Cumulative Effect causes most degenerative disease and that the Cumulative Effect is a result of the combination of toxins accumulating in the body, impaired cell regeneration and a weakened immune system. Your immune system is your primary defense against the bodily breakdowns resulting from the modern lifestyle. If toxins accumulate in your body or your body begins to break down at a molecular level and you have no defense against their side effects, you are incredibly vulnerable to disease.

Therefore, the frequency, severity and duration of the colds and flu that one gets is a good measure of how one's immune system reacts to more serious threats like synthetic chemicals, toxins and genetic defects like cancer. In other words, people who are frequently sick are the most susceptible to getting degenerative disease because their immune systems are incapable of fighting the cellular defects that result from living in the modern world (all of which is a function of unhealthy habits). If you are one of these people, you are at the highest risk of sitting across from your doctor some day soon listening to the words, "We're not sure what causes …" If you are one of the people in the middle group, the ones that get sick two to three times per year, you are also at a risk of chronic disease over time. Your immune system is doing an average job of protecting you, but that is not enough in the modern context. If you are one of the very few people in the fist group that rarely gets sick, you are at lower risk and you need to help the people you love learn to follow your habits so they can have a vigorously healthy immune system!

Your immune system is the only doctor that is chemically equipped to repair your body from all of the toxins and cellular damage that you inevitably encounter in our world. Therefore, the best defense against sickness and disease is not a defense at all. It's a good *offense*: following healthy habits in order to develop a strong immune system.

Immune-Centered Health
In my opinion and my experience, healthy habits are the key to fighting the epidemic of chronic illness and disease facing mankind. This is because they bolster the immune system, our only real defense against the sophisticated illnesses we see overtaking our friends and family. I am not confident that science will advance enough to develop effective cures for life-threatening chronic illnesses and degenerative diseases in our lifetime. The best that we can hope to see from medical science in our lifetimes are more and more targeted symptom treatments (because symptoms are scientifically easier to isolate than causes). And since symptom treatments typically don't do anything about the causes of our sickness and because they are only useful once you get sick, we have only ourselves, our habits and our immune systems to rely on to defend us against getting sick in the first place.
A healthy immune system can fortify you to fight the epidemic of disease because it is by far the most complete and effective weapon available to combat sickness. A healthy immune system protects us with:

- An extensive security force: The immune system is a functional system with glands, nodes and tissue interconnected and spread around the body. This acts like a series of spies spread over vast territory, watching out for foreign invaders (antigens).

- An early response system: As soon as an antigen enters or develops inside your body, such as a mutated cell or a virus cell, it will come into contact with cells of the immune system. Instantly, the immune system goes on high alert and begins production of a specific weapon to fight the antigen based on its unique characteristics.

- An endless arsenal of specific weapons: The immune system produces antibodies that are specifically designed to seek out, attack and neutralize any "non-self" antigen that it has detected. It is believed that the immune system can develop an antibody to fight any form of antigen.

- Non-stop, tireless fighting: Once an antigen is detected, the immune system fights the foreign invaders with targeted weapons nonstop, day and night until the antigen is neutralized.

Because we live in highly synthetic surroundings in the West, we take in large quantities of a vast array of toxins every day simply by eating, drinking, breathing and touching things. In most cases, those toxins are recognized as "non-self" by your immune system and the series of defense steps described above goes into effect. If you live in the "modern world," at any given moment in time, your immune system is probably fighting an assortment of antigens with a range of antibodies.

A well-functioning immune system is a prerequisite to survive in a world of synthetic toxins with untold molecular side effects. Poorly functioning immune systems are not able to rally as quickly or neutralize antigens as completely. Poor nutrition, dehydration, lack of proper rest and an overload of stress can weaken the body's ability fight. As a result, toxins have a chance to accumulate in the body, damaging cells and tissue.

Eventually, this damage and the inability to produce healthy cells erode the systems of the body to the point that irreversible chronic disease sets in.

The immune system, not drug-centered medicine, should be viewed as your primary weapon in the fight against sickness. Immune-centered health works from the premise that the body can heal itself if given the chance. Instead of relying on doctors, pills and shots to keep you healthy, cultivate your immune system by following habits of health. It is far more capable of protecting you than the medical community is. In the (less likely) event that you do get sick and need the help of medicine, choose treatments that are the least harmful and most likely to create a healing response from your body. They should be designed to facilitate healing by knocking down the illness to a level that can be managed by the immune system.

As you will read, there are very explicit things that you can (and must) do to promote your body's healing system. The influences that improve or reduce the effectiveness of the human immune system are very specific, but they are not simple events. A healthy immune system is based on the choices that you make every day, or, more specifically, the habits that you follow and the influences those habits have on your body.

The Choice
Previously, I was a sickly person. I was sick all of the time – colds, flu, pink eye, ear and sinus infections, stomach viruses, etc. I was tired all of the time and had weird skin rashes and random nose bleeds. I had strange digestive difficulties and unusual sleeping problems. I was not healthy and I was degenerating year after year. My body was so run down that I developed cancer at the ripe old age of 18. Even after doctors poisoned my cancer away, my habits remained the same and I continued to degenerate year after year, sicker and sicker and sicker.

Now I know that all of these conditions, even the cancer, were symptoms of the same central cause. My health had been degenerating as a result of my unhealthy habits and The Cumulative Effect was showing up all over my body. I took responsibility for my health, educated myself, studied the healthiest people in the world, and, through trial and error, I adopted their habits.

Of course there are no more tumors, but even the subtler signs of my sickness are now gone. Now that I have adopted Habits of Health, all of the signs of my sickness have disappeared. I don't get colds, flu, diarrhea, and rashes. I no longer have bloody noses and dry cracking skin. I require less sleep, I am more alert, I easily maintain a healthy weight, and I have more energy. I don't miss work, I'm not a hypochondriac, I don't have to take side-effect causing medicines, and I don't spend the money that I used to spend on doctors and drugs.

I now have a calm confidence, if not bravado, about my health. Those subconscious worries about developing an incurable disease and dying young or being a sickly, bed-ridden old man are gone. I am confident that I will live a long, healthy, productive life. So long, in fact, that I have had to modify my worries (like most, I can still find something to worry about). I now worry that I will outlive my retirement savings. I am 38 years old and I feel that there is a good chance that I will live long enough to see all three of my young children retire.

Based on my research and my own experiences, I now believe that most people living today will suffer from multiple chronic illnesses and/or diseases that they can prevent from ever happening. I believe that the world in which we live, breath, eat, drink, play, learn and work can easily tear down the health of a human being. If you are one of those people who assume that you will be among the very, very few who live a life of unhealthy habits and avoid chronic illness and disease altogether, you are being incredibly immature and you know it. Just look at the statistics in Part 1 of this book. Don't take my word for it – look around at your family and friends. If you live a life of unhealthy habits for 20, 30, 40 years, you will develop one or more chronic illnesses. You can take that to the bank.

If you are reading this book, you obviously care about your health. You are investing time into this book because you are/were sick, someone you care about is/was sick or because you fear the inevitability of sickness for you and your loved ones. In any of these cases, you have three alternatives among which you must choose. You can put off making a choice, but don't put it off too long. Not choosing is still making a choice.

Alternative #1. Trust conventional medicine. Most people believe that traditional medicine will keep them healthy. The medical industry's intense focus on improving the *survival rate* of disease instead of reducing the *incidence rate* of disease highlights its emphasis on disease treatment (sick care) instead of disease prevention. Therefore, putting your trust in the medical industry is essentially committing yourself to disease and *hoping* that the treatment options that are available will allow you to enjoy a reasonable quality of life while you postpone your date with the reaper.

As the author Rick Page says, *hope is not a strategy*. In particular, hope is not a strategy when it comes to trusting your health to sick care. I believe that the immaturity of our science prevents us from knowing more than 20% of what we need to know about the human body in order to create effective treatments. Treatment options typically revolve around pharmaceutical drugs to suppress the symptoms of illness and virtually all drugs have a litany of side effects. And if treatment drugs cannot yet be tailored to complete a specific mission in the body without impacting other systems and creating side effects, isn't it *impossible* for medical science to create cures that counteract degenerative diseases resulting from a complex interaction spanning many of the body's various systems?

Let me say this again because it is an important point: The long-term presence of various toxins in the body alongside the continuous degradation of the body's life-sustaining systems results in damage at the cellular and molecular level across many of the body's systems (the Cumulative Effect) and ultimately results in degenerative disease (cancer, arthritis, heart disease, dementia…). If medical science is only advanced enough to create drugs that eliminate a specific symptom in the body (headache, high blood pressure, joint pain, etc.) but, in the process, quite clumsily cause a host of unintended consequences to other areas of the body (side effects), how could it create drugs to cure (eliminate) complex diseases that span multiple systems of the body?

Putting your hope for health in sick care is like putting a nine-year old in charge of your life savings. It might work, but chances are it won't.

Alternative #2. Trust your health to silver bullets. The majority of what we read, see and hear about health would have us believe that there are quick fixes for any health problem. The pharmaceutical industry, the supplement industry, the fitness industry, many alternative health practitioners, the health and beauty industry and the consumer products industry all want the consumer to believe that the remedy to what ails him is within their products and services.

In most cases, it *is* too good to be true and your subconscious has been telling you that all along. The little voice inside your head tells you every time you see one of those silly infomercials or obnoxious ads. Your heart wants to believe that you can prevent sickness with a quick fix, but you know in your head that human health is far too sophisticated and complex. Our hearts want to believe that Juan Ponce de León did find a fountain of youth in Florida, but our heads know that it's just a tall tale.

Are the companies behind these products lying? Well yes, sadly they are. But in a for-profit business, it is called "marketing." Maybe that sounds harsh to you. Maybe you think that is too broad a brush. But ask yourself this: if any of the quick fix, silver bullets really repaired a broken body (any of the vast arrays of exotic supplements, for example), would we have the epidemic of disease that we are facing today?

There is no magic pill, no magic potion and no book of *real* cures that the government doesn't want you to know about. There is no miracle cream, no rainforest remedy and no super-nutrient that can fix your health once it is broken. The truth is that human health is sophisticated. It is complex to screw up and, once it is broken, it is complex to fix.

Alternative #3. Adopt healthy habits. The developed world is fantastically advanced in its ability to react. The medical system in the developed world is very efficient at managing trauma and treating diseases *once they occur.* This "act-in-response" approach in medicine has resulted in a reactive mindset when it comes to all aspects of human health. After years of unhealthy living, when someone has a health problem, they make a change in their habits: reacting to a stroke by eating better, reacting to a heart attack by starting an exercise program, or reacting to high blood pressure by changing their diet, for example.

Yet millions and millions of people suffer from disease, spend the later years of their lives without their dignity, and die well before their time. Why? Because "act-in-response" management of health is not effective at keeping us well.

Health is more like automobile maintenance. You have to regularly take actions to maintain your car – washing it, changing the oil, checking the tire pressure, replacing the power steering fluid, checking the tightness of the belts, watching for tread wear, etc. If you don't, things break down and they are dangerous, expensive and time consuming to repair.

Your health is the same. You have to regularly take actions to maintain your health – eating right, getting the right amount of clean water, being active, avoiding dangerous chemicals, getting plenty of sleep, etc. If you don't, things break down and they are dangerous, expensive and time consuming to repair (*if* they can be repaired).
People are proactive about automobile maintenance. This is mostly a result of the schedule provided by the manufacturer and the profit motivation of the service departments and auto repair shops. These things, along with conscientious, well trained consumers, create the infrastructure to reinforce proactive automobile maintenance.

Like automobile maintenance, health maintenance should be proactive. Yet, there is no manufacturer's maintenance schedule that comes with the human body. And there are no repair shops running commercials to remind you to maintain your health. Also, people are generally not conscientious or well "trained" when it comes to being proactive about their health. So, in order for people to be proactive about maintaining their health, they need an "infrastructure" to remind them to take the correct actions. This is why habits are so powerful.

Habits create an artificial support and reminder system. Once a set of actions is adopted as a habit, the body recognizes the pattern and accepts it as "normal." When the adopted set of actions is not performed at the expected interval, the human body expects the stimulus provided by the habit and physically yearns for it. It literally craves it. This support system is the "infrastructure" that we humans need to remind us to proactively maintain our health. It is the body's built in reminder system and we can program that reminder system to prompt us to consistently do things that promote our health.

The adoption of healthy habits is the only way to ensure that there is a consistent, positive force supporting your health. In a world that constantly pulls us toward an unhealthy lifestyle, healthy habits are the only way to guard yourself against life's many health risks. The world around us provides too many unhealthy opportunities to ignore. When you do stumble and skip that workout or eat an unhealthy meal, your re-trained mind and body will crave the stimulus of your healthy habits and pull you back to them. You will have reprogrammed your mind and body to work to your benefit, to stand guard for your health. For the person that is concerned about his health, it is the only realistic preventative health approach.

I wish that I could live a life of reckless abandon and know that the medical industry could repair whatever breaks down in me. I wish there was a book with secret cures that *really* worked that the FDA didn't want me to know about. I wish there was an exotic rainforest fruit that could cure disease. I wish there were a pill that we could all take that would prevent degenerative diseases.

Our hearts hope that someone or something else will take care of us, but our head knows better. Resilient health, it turns out, is not found in a pill, powder or potion. It is not found in a physician's office. Our health is in our hands, not someone or something else's. Our habits determine our health.

PART II

The Eight Habits of Healthy People

When it comes to their health, people seem to generally know what they should and should not do, but they seem to have a hard time turning their abundant knowledge about health into action. They can't convert their nagging conscience into a lifestyle that keeps them healthy.

Habits of health are the link between health knowledge and health action. They enable us to convert our nagging conscience into a set of right actions that get consistently applied. They cause us to regularly do the things that we know we need to do and can't do by force of will and memory alone.

The eight habits in Part Two of this book are the habits that form a healthy lifestyle. They are *the* habits of health and they can and will keep you healthy. If you follow these habits, you will reduce the Cumulative Effect on your body, your health will improve, and you will considerably reduce your chances of developing any kind of chronic illness. I am living proof.

I spent over twenty years researching health. I read, viewed, listened to, attended, and tried just about everything available on preventative health. My research and experimentation spanned traditional medicine, alternative medicine, nutrition, fitness, faith healing and many truly bizarre branches of *alternative* alternative health.

I didn't set out to write a book. I simply wanted to improve my own health and reduce the chances that I would again face a deadly chronic disease. I was so motivated to get healthy that I tried nearly every recommendation that I came across. There were so many recommendations that I had to start qualifying them before I would try a new one. I began to keep a journal in which I categorized health recommendations based on the frequency with which the recommendation came up in my research, the consistency of the recommendation across my research, and the perceived impact that the recommendation had on my health and the health of the people recommending and using it. Interestingly, over the course of several years, I found that the recommendations of this broad group of health experts fell into ten categories of related recommendations. To my surprise, there was great similarity in the recommendations of these seemingly contradictory fields of health. As I studied the recommendations, one category began to look awfully similar to another, and ten collapsed into nine and then nine collapsed into eight. I experimented with these recommendations, ultimately refining them into eight specific habits that I adopted as a part of my lifestyle.

To make a long story short, I became *incredibly* healthy. The best way to describe my health improvement, as I have said earlier, is that I went from being a person who got four to six lingering colds per year to a person who got three or four colds in five years. In the space of time that I would have typically gotten 20 to 30 lingering colds, I got three or four. If that is not an *incredible* improvement in health, I can't imagine what is.

And that is just one measure of my health. I am healthier in so many other ways. I sleep more restfully, I have more energy, my mind is sharper, my memory is better, my skin and hair are healthier, cuts and scrapes heal faster, I have fewer injuries from physical activity, and I feel better in so many other ways. I also know that this level of health is preventing the return of degenerative disease in my body. If I am able to fight off the colds and flu that I am sure I still come into contact with, then I am certain that my body is fighting off toxins and cellular malfunctions that could lead to degenerative disease in my body.

One March afternoon while sitting alone on the beach in Puerto Rico reading one of the latest gimmick health books and pondering my own health, I realized a few things. I knew that I wanted the same kind of health I had achieved for my family and friends, but I knew most of them would never do the research and experimentation that I had done. I also knew that no one would listen to me if I tried to tell them what I had learned.

And in that moment, on that beach, I realized that I had to write a book. I realized that it was my duty to share what I knew about health, and, quite frankly, I knew writing a book was the only way people would take me seriously.

Based upon my research, there are eight habits that determine the Cumulative Effect in a person's body. Each of the eight chapters that follow includes the lessons I have learned about applying the individual habits. And, in each chapter, I provide some hints on easy ways to get started with each habit.

When you read the following eight chapters, don't spend time worrying about how you can make these habits part of your life. And don't be discouraged if you've tried to make one of these habits part of your life before and failed. In Part III of this book, I will share with you a simple approach for habit adoption that anyone can follow. Read these chapters with the goal of gaining and enhancing your health knowledge. In Part III, you will learn how to convert that health knowledge into consistent health actions.

Chapter 5

Live on Nature's Harvest

What we eat may affect our risk for several of the leading causes of death for Americans, notably, coronary heart disease, stroke, atherosclerosis, diabetes, and some types of cancer. These disorders together now account for more than two-thirds of all deaths in the United States.
Dr. C. Everett Koop, former U.S. Surgeon General

I recently stayed in a hotel in downtown Boston, Massachusetts, and needed to arrange an early breakfast before catching a flight back to my home in Atlanta. Hanging on the doorknob inside my room was the ubiquitous breakfast order card containing a handful of breakfast meal choices, some a la carte items and lines for my name, room number and desired delivery time. Once completed, the cards are hung on the outside doorknob and collected by the room service fairy some time during the night. I suppose that having these cards in advance allows the kitchen to prepare your food throughout the night with a small staff instead of having to staff the kitchen en masse in the morning when a flood of calls comes rolling in, but I digress.

This breakfast order card was almost identical to the hundreds of other order cards that I have filled out over the years. However, this time I noticed something that I had never really paid attention to in the past, which was the content and names of the breakfast meals: The Continental Breakfast, The Sunrise Breakfast, The Healthy Start Breakfast and The American Breakfast. The names are almost universal, but the content varies by hotel. However, it occurred to me that morning that the content of one of these breakfasts never seemed to vary like the others. One of these breakfasts always has the same unhealthy combination of eggs, hash browns, your choice of bacon sausage or ham, and toast with butter and jelly. Can you guess which of the four breakfasts this was? Of course you can. It was the American Breakfast.

We have a national eating disorder in the United States. We obsess over health and nutrition and yet we are the unhealthiest nation in the world when it comes to what we eat. The typical American diet contains excessive amounts of fat, sugar and salt and a significant lack of fiber.

To make matters worse, we have wild swings of popular nutritional opinion from one decade to the next – avoid saturated fat, replace saturated fat with hydrogenated fat, limit carbohydrates, eliminate hydrogenated fat, eat whole grain, etc.

Recently, the U.S. federal government has encouraged Americans to increase their consumption of plant foods such as fruits, vegetables and grains. This is a result of a growing body of evidence that they offer more health benefits that previously understood, including possibly contributing to the prevention of heart disease and certain types of cancer. For example, one recent study found that people who eat fruits and vegetables more than three times per day reduce their risk of having a stroke or dying from cardiovascular disease by nearly 25% compared to those who eat them less than once per day, on average. However, only about 10% of adults and 15% of children in the U.S. meet the government's recommendation for daily fruit and vegetable consumption. As a result, many people are suffering from nutritional deficiencies even though they are getting plenty of calories and may be overweight.

It is believed that the consumption of plant foods improves human health because of the availability of beneficial nutrients inside of them. The human body replaces 95% of its living cells every year with new ones, and a diet rich in plant foods ensures that the newly produced cells have the nutrients available to be healthy ones. If you are under-nourished or have DNA damaged by toxic buildup in the body or by oxidation, you will reproduce unhealthy cells. With 95% of your cells being replaced every year, it does not take long for your body to become degenerated. Therefore, it is critical, at all stages of life, to nourish your body with the appropriate foods.

Many people living in undeveloped areas of the world do not have access to the high fat/sugar/ salt diets that developed nations like the United States enjoy and therefore exist on nature's harvest alone. One such group on the island of Kitava off of the coast of Papua New Guinea was studied in a report published in 1993. In the study, it was found that Kitavans had an almost nonexistent rate of cardiac disease and stroke despite the fact that nearly 80% of the population smoked tobacco (that they grew themselves). While this is not a license to eat healthy so that you can resume the awful habit of smoking, it does seem to indicate that a healthy diet interacts with other habits, good and bad, to protect our health.

The top ten causes of insurance claims and hospitalization in the United States in 1990 included cancer, hear attacks, diabetes, obesity, hemorrhoids, diverticulitis, diverticulosis, peptic ulcer, hiatal hernia, appendicitis and gall stones. According to Jordan Rubin, author of *The Maker's Diet*, these conditions rarely occur among primitive cultures living around the world today. "Of course, other factors figure in our picture health as well – genetics, environmental toxins, lifestyle choices, emotional and mental factors, and cultural trends that affect health – but diet remains the single most influential factor in overall human health."

The further that a food is from a whole, natural food, the unhealthier it is for our bodies. Because food is chemically altered during processing, the more that we refine and process a food, the more we destroy its nutrition and inherent healthful qualities. To properly nourish your body, half or more of your food should be fresh, raw, living food. That is, it should be uncooked, unprocessed, unpreserved, unflavored fruits, vegetables, nuts, grains and seeds.

Fruits and Vegetables
Over many thousands of years, fruits and vegetables developed on the earth alongside humans, so, it makes sense that their chemical makeup supports our nutritional needs better than man-made or man-modified foods. Fruits and vegetables are naturally low in fat and calories and contain no cholesterol. They are important sources of many nutrients including potassium, folate (folic acid), vitamin A, vitamin E, and vitamin C, and they are loaded with fiber. In my opinion, they are the best form of preventative medicine that we can put into our bodies.

Studies suggest that people who eat more vegetables and fruits have a lower risk for some types of cancer including lung, oral, esophageal, prostate and colon cancer. And, according to the Prostate Cancer Foundation, men are 30% less likely to develop prostate cancer if they eat lycopene-rich cooked tomato products regularly (like tomato sauce, tomato soup and ketchup) and 20% less likely to develop the disease if they regularly eat cruciferous vegetables (broccoli, cabbage, cauliflower, kale and Brussels sprouts).

A recent cancer study at the University of California San Diego found that fruits and vegetables reduced overall cancer risk. The study, published in the September 2005 issue of the journal *Cancer, Epidemiology, Biomarkers and Prevention*, found that cancer risk was reduced by roughly 50% in subjects eating nine servings of fruits and vegetables compared to subjects eating only five servings, and those eating five servings had a 50% lower risk of developing cancer than those eating only two servings of fruits and vegetables.

In addition, eating more fruits and vegetables can help reduce three of the major risk factors for heart attack: high cholesterol, high blood pressure and excess body weight. Fruit and vegetable consumption also helps reduce the risk of stroke because heart disease and high blood pressure are major risk factors for stroke. In one of the most comprehensive studies to date, The Nurse's Health Study, 110,000 men and women had their health habits followed for 14 years. The study found that the higher the intake of fruits and vegetables, the lower the incidence of cardiovascular disease. In fact, those who averaged eight or more servings per day of fruits and vegetables were 30% less likely to get cardiovascular disease than those who ate only 1.5 servings per day.

In response to all of this new health information, the U.S. Departments of Health and Human Services and Agriculture updated their Dietary Guidelines for Americans in 2005. The previous version of the guidelines, published in 2000, recommended that adults eat five to nine servings of fruits and vegetables per day. In the 2005 version, nutrition recommendations are based on a person's gender, age and physical activity, but the recommended servings increased to seven to thirteen.

What counts as a serving?

Fruits
- 1 medium apple, banana or orange
- ½ cup of chopped, cooked, or canned fruit
- ¾ cup of 100% fruit juice

Vegetables
- 1 cup of raw, leafy vegetables
- ½ cup of other cooked or raw vegetables, chopped,
- ¾ cup of 100% vegetable juice

Consuming seven to thirteen servings of fruits and vegetables per day can be a challenge and it is not just because of our fast-paced lifestyle or the abundance of alternative food choices available to us. It is also because seven to thirteen servings *is a lot* if you have a diet that has been built around the wrong types of food. Many people are accustomed to seeing their shopping carts and dinner plates full of the wrong types and wrong proportions of food. In general, people have over-bought and over-consumed things like meats, snack foods and sweets for so long that it takes some time to get used to buying and consuming the right types of foods in the right amounts. At the end of this chapter, you will find a load of great recommendations on how to get more servings of plant foods into your diet. For now, just remember that you simply cannot eat too many fruits and vegetables.

In eating all those fruits and vegetables that your body needs to remain healthy, it turns out that variety may be just as important as quantity. Simply eating seven bananas per day is not quite what the doctor ordered! You have to eat a variety of fruits and vegetables to really get all of the benefits.

A century ago, tens of thousands of crop varieties were cultivated and eaten around the world. Today, potatoes, corn and peas make up 40% of the vegetables consumed by Americans. Throw in soybeans and tomatoes and these five vegetables make up the vast majority of the vegetables eaten in the West.

There are over 12,000 phytonutrients (enzymes, vitamins, minerals, etc.) in any given fruit or vegetable and they vary considerably from vegetable to vegetable and from fruit to fruit. Phytonutrients appear to protect the body against the damage to tissues that occurs constantly as a result of normal metabolism. They are found in the pigment of plants such as carotenes and carotenoids (red, pink and orange plants), chlorophyll (green plants) and flavonoids (berries). Lycopene, mentioned above as being linked to the reduction of prostate cancer incidence, is a carotenoid phytonutrient found in the pigment of tomatoes, carrots, watermelon and pink grapefruit. Cruciferous vegetables – broccoli, cabbage, cauliflower, radishes, kale, Brussels sprouts, collard greens and mustard greens – contain more phytonutrients with anticancer properties than any other group of fruits or vegetables. There are hundreds of different phytonutrients in fruits and vegetables that protect and heal our bodies.

When a person's fruit and vegetable intake is limited, he may never get the protective benefits of many important phytonutrients. Color is one important way to ensure that you are getting a variety of phytonutrients in your diet. Strive to get as many colors in your daily consumption of fruits and vegetables as possible:

- Phytonutrients and vitamins found in green fruits and vegetables like broccoli, honeydew melon, cucumbers and cabbage sharpen eyesight, strengthen bones and fight birth defects.
- Phytonutrients in yellow and orange fruits and vegetables like oranges, carrots, cantaloupes, sweet potatoes and yellow bell peppers reduce risk for certain cancers, boost immune function and protect your eyes and heart.
- Phytonutrients in red fruits and vegetables like tomatoes, grapefruit, red grapes, red bell peppers and cherries lower the risk for prostate cancer, protect the heart and the memory.
- Phytonutrients found in blue and purple fruits and vegetables like blueberries, purple grapes, eggplant and raisins provide an extraordinarily high amount of anti-oxidants to protect against oxidation in the body.

My staple vegetables are broccoli, cucumber, tomato, carrots and spinach and my staple fruits are grapes, bananas and apples. If I am not intentional about seeking out different foods, I wind up with the same things week after week, which limits the range of phytonutrients in my diet. I have found that the best way to get variety is to force myself to try something new every time I buy produce. Bring home cauliflower instead of broccoli. Try plantains instead of bananas. Get peaches and pears instead of apples. And it doesn't always have to be a completely new food. It could simply be a different variety of the same fruit or vegetable. Try yellow bell peppers instead of green or red next week. Try Granny Smith apples instead of Fuji.

Consuming more servings and a wider variety of fruits in vegetables takes some intentionality, I have found, and while eating fruits and vegetables fresh and raw is the best, you should strive to eat them in any form as often as you can. Be mindful when storing your fresh fruits and vegetables though. As a fresh-picked fruit ages on your shelf, it is losing its vitamin and mineral content. Make sure to refrigerate or freeze your fresh fruits and vegetables to maintain their healthy state for as long as possible. Store-bought frozen fruits and vegetables, it turns out, can actually be more nutritious than fresh ones because they are often picked ripe and quickly frozen, locking in their nutrients at the peak state of their health.

Cooking and processing can also reduce the nutritional content of fruits and vegetables. Boiling vegetables, especially for long periods, can leach out their content of water-soluble (B and C) vitamins. Microwaving and steaming are the best cooking methods to use in order to preserve the nutritional content of vegetables. Because of the high heat used in the canning process, canned fruits and vegetables have reduced levels of heat-sensitive and water-soluble nutrients. Also, be aware that some fruits are packed in heavy syrup (sugar), and some canned vegetables are high in sodium and fat.

However you do it, simply eat more fruits and vegetables. And when you do, try to eat a wide array of colors. Fruits and vegetables are the best preventative medicine known to man.

Grains, Nuts, Seeds and Beans
Grains, nuts and beans are also important contributors to health. Like fruits and vegetables, they are full of nutrition. Also like fruits and vegetables, these important foods are under-appreciated and under-consumed by those with access to more processed food choices.

Grains may be the most misunderstood healthy food, largely because grains are the most marketed basic ingredient of many staple foods. "Whole grain" is heavily marketed because it is an important source of many nutrients including dietary fiber, several B vitamins (thiamin, riboflavin, niacin, and folate), and minerals (iron, magnesium, and selenium). In addition, it has been linked to the reduction of the risk of heart disease and certain cancers.

A whole grain is made up of three parts: the bran, endosperm and germ. Refined grains are made from the endosperm. Because the bran and germ contain much of the vitamins, minerals and all of the fiber found in grains, whole grains have more fiber and nutrients than refined (or processed) grains. Whole grains include brown rice, buckwheat, bulgur (cracked wheat), oatmeal, popcorn, whole wheat cereals, muesli, whole grain barley, whole grain cornmeal, whole rye, whole wheat bread, whole wheat crackers, whole wheat pasta, whole wheat sandwich buns and rolls, whole wheat tortillas and wild rice. Refined grains include cornbread, corn tortillas, couscous, crackers, flour tortillas, grits, noodles, pasta, pitas, pretzels, most ready-to-eat breakfast cereals, corn flakes, white bread, white sandwich buns and rolls and white rice.

Always read ingredient lists carefully to see if the product you are buying contains whole grain. Ingredient lists can be misleading and it is not an accident. For example, while bran provides fiber, products with added bran or bran alone (for example, oat bran) are not necessarily whole grain products. Foods labeled with the words "multi-grain," "stone-ground," "100% wheat," "cracked wheat," "seven-grain,"

What counts as a serving?
• 1 slice of bread
• ½ cup of cooked cereal, pasta or rice
• 1 ounce of ready-to-eat cereal
• 1 cup of flaked cereal
• ¼ cup of nugget-type cereal
• ½ cup of nuts
• ½ cup of cooked dry beans
• 2 tablespoons of peanut butter

or "bran" are usually not whole-grain products. Color is not an indication of a whole grain either. Bread can be brown because of molasses or other added ingredients.

While whole grain is a great source of many nutrients and an important part of a healthy diet, it is not a great source of protein. Nuts are, though. In addition to being one of the best plant sources of protein, they are rich in fiber, phytonutrients and antioxidants such as Vitamin E and selenium. Nuts are also high in fat - but mostly monounsaturated and polyunsaturated fats (the good fats). In addition, they contain fiber and antioxidants, which could lower your risk of heart disease.

Researchers found that people who eat nuts regularly have lower risks of heart disease. In 1996, the Iowa Women's Healthy Study found that women who ate nuts more than four times a week were 40% less likely to die of heart disease. Two years later, another study conducted by the Harvard School of Public Health found a similar result in another group of women subjects. Potential heart health benefits of nuts were also found among men. In 2002, the Physician's Health Study found that men who consumed nuts two or more times per week had reduced risks of sudden cardiac death.

The type of nut you eat isn't that important. Walnuts, almonds, hazelnuts, you name it – almost every type of nut has a lot of nutrition packed into a tiny package. Walnuts are one of the best-studied nuts, and it's been shown they contain high amounts of omega-3 fatty acids. Almonds, macadamia nuts, hazelnuts and pecans are other nuts that appear to be quite heart healthy. Even peanuts – which are technically not a nut, but a legume – seem to be relatively healthy.

There is growing evidence that people who eat nuts regularly tend to live longer and the same is also true of beans. This is probably because, according to the United Stated Department of Agriculture, analyses show that people who eat beans consume more vitamins and minerals than individuals who don't eat beans. Dry beans and other pulses, also referred to as legumes (navy, red, black, kidney and white beans; cowpeas and black-eye peas; lentils and split peas; fava and lima beans; etc) are nutrient-dense. That is, calorie for calorie, beans supply high levels of various nutrients. A single serving of beans supplies loads of complex carbohydrates and fiber and they are a good source of B vitamins including folic acid. Beans also provide the minerals iron, potassium, selenium, magnesium and even some calcium. Beans provide little fat and absolutely no cholesterol. Eating beans regularly may help lower risk of colon cancer, reduce blood cholesterol (a leading cause of heart disease) and lower the risk diabetes.

Beans, nuts, seeds and whole grains are among nature's healthiest foods. The same general rule of thumb applies to these foods as to fruits and vegetables: you can't eat too much of them. The government's dietary guidelines for Americans suggest consuming eight to ten servings of grains every day with at least half of them being whole grains (see serving size chart above). Serving recommendations for nuts, seeds and beans are not quite as clear cut, primarily because the government groups them with meat due to their protein content. Generally, the dietary guidelines for Americans recommend eating five to six "ounce equivalents" daily from the meat group (an ounce equivalent is 1 ounce of meat, poultry or fish, ¼ cup cooked dry beans, 1 egg, 1 tablespoon of peanut butter, or ½ ounce of nuts). Most Americans over-consume meat so the government guidelines probably under-emphasize the importance of nuts, seeds and beans. Instead of trying to count servings, my recommendation for consuming whole grain, nuts, seeds and beans is just like my recommendation for fruits and vegetables: eat more of them by replacing unhealthy processed foods, sweets and some of your meats with them.

What about Meat, Dairy, Poultry and Fish?

The human body needs protein. Proteins function as the building blocks for bones, muscles, cartilage, skin, and blood. They are also the building blocks for enzymes, hormones, and vitamins. Unfortunately, the modern diet in most Western nations contains far too much protein. Most adults in the Western world eat about 100 grams of protein per day, or about twice what their bodies need, and most of the excess protein in the Western diet comes from the over-consumption of meat.

The conspiracy theorist in me, of course, believes that the meat

> What is a vegetarian and what is a vegan?
>
> Vegetarian diets differ in composition, although all avoid red meat. Strict vegetarian diets that avoid all animal products, including milk and eggs are often called *vegan* diets. Vegetarian and vegan diets include many health-promoting features; they tend to be low in saturated fats and high in fiber, vitamins, and phytochemicals. A vegetarian or vegan diet can be quite healthful if it is carefully planned and provides adequate calories and protein. However, diets including lean meats in small to moderate amounts can be just as healthful.

marketers promoted the idea that we "need some protein in our stomachs" in order to function properly. (How many times have you heard Mom say that?) Over time, meats have become the main course at lunch and dinner and beans, vegetables, fruits, etc. (if there are any included in the meal) are the side dishes.

Meat is not, by itself, inherently bad. The saturated fat in the meat is what is bad for you, and it is bad for two specific reasons. First, diets that are high in animal (saturated) fats raise "bad" cholesterol levels in the blood. The "bad" cholesterol is called LDL (low-density lipoprotein) cholesterol. High LDL cholesterol, in turn, increases the risk for coronary heart disease.

Second, diets that are high in animal fats tend to increase your exposure to harmful toxins. With such widespread use of pesticides and antibiotics in farming, animals like cows, pigs, chickens and turkeys ingest significant amounts of these and other industrial toxins. These toxins are stored in their fatty tissues, which you eat (more on this later). Therefore, unless it is organic, the fattier the cut of meat you eat, the more toxins you take in to your body. In addition, some studies have linked eating large amounts of preserved meat to increased risk of colorectal and stomach cancers. This association may be due to nitrites, which are added to many lunch meats, hams and hot dogs to maintain color and to prevent contamination with bacteria.

To reduce your intake of harmful animal fat, limit fatty cuts of beef, pork, lamb, regular ground beef (75% to 85% lean), regular sausages, hot dogs, bacon and luncheon meats such as bologna and salami. The leanest cuts of beef are the filet, tenderloin, cuts with the words "loin" or "round" in the name (round eye, top round, bottom round, round tip, top loin, and top sirloin), chuck shoulder and arm roasts. Also, choose extra lean ground beef. The label should say at least "90% lean," and you may be able to find ground beef that is 93% or 95% lean. The cut of chicken and turkey that contains the least amount of fat is the breast, without the skin. Other good choices include lean cuts of buffalo, lamb, venison, goose and duck. Also, for you grill lovers (and I'm one of you by the way), charred meats have been found to contain a highly carcinogenic substance called benzopyrene. To enjoy grilled meats, instead of placing the meat directly over the charcoal, cook using the indirect method placing the meat away from the charcoal. This method takes longer, but it is far safer for your health and the taste of the meat, in my opinion, is better.

I also recommend buying organic meat. The healthiest meat and poultry products to buy are labeled "certified organic free range." This means that the animals graze unconfined in fields not treated with industrial chemicals like insecticides and herbicides and they are not treated with man-made drugs like antibiotics. Also, to avoid the high levels of metals such as mercury and other toxins such as PCB's commonly found in some fish, buy wild caught (not farm-raised), cold water fish. Safe, wild caught fish choices include Anchovies, Arctic char, Pacific flounder, herring, Pacific sole, tilapia, Alaska and Pacific salmon, striped bass, red snapper, orange roughy and cod. You will pay more for the unpolluted meat, poultry and fish products (which always strikes me as a bit ironic), but your health is worth it.

Don't forget that animal fat is in all animal products including milk and dairy products. Fat-free, 1/2% fat and 1% fat milk all provide the same nutrients as whole milk and 2% fat milk, but they are much lower in fat, saturated fatty acids, cholesterol, calories and harmful pesticides. There are skim milk alternatives for milk, cheese, butter, cream, ice cream, chocolate, etc. Use fat-free, ½% fat or 1% fat organic milk and nonfat or low-fat organic dairy products. If you're used to whole-milk products, you may find it easier to make the change slowly to lower-fat foods. Try 1% fat milk first. Then when you're used to that, move to 1/2% fat milk. This will make it much easier if you decide to ultimately change to fat-free milk.

The Standard American Diet (S.A.D.) tends to be built around high-fat animal products. Instead, the human diet should be built around vegetables, fruits, beans, seeds and grains with animal products as a garnish or side dish like our ancestors' diets were. Beans, peas, nuts, and seeds are also good sources of protein and many other nutrients including B vitamins (niacin, thiamin, riboflavin, and B6), vitamin E, iron, zinc, and magnesium. When you do eat meat, select low fat meats and include fish in meals in order to reduce your cholesterol and your exposure to harmful toxins.

As stated above, the government's dietary guidelines suggest consuming five to six "ounce equivalents" from the meat, beans, nuts and seeds food group per day. It is recommended that you eat this in three ounce

> **What is a three ounce equivalent?**
> - Two ¼ inch thin slices of lean roast beef
> - Chicken leg with thigh (no skin)
> - ¾ cup cooked dry beans
> - 3 medium eggs
> - 3 tablespoons of peanut butter
> - 1½ ounces of nuts or seeds

equivalent portions. That's really all the lean meat, poultry or fish your body needs. And remember when choosing your meats that most fish and poultry have fewer calories than fatty cuts of red meat. They do contain cholesterol, though, so keep portions the same as for red meat.

What's the Deal with Fat?
"One fat, two fats, good fats, bad fats. Should I eat those silly trans fats? Mono fats, poly fats, saturated and Omega fats. Which are the good and bad fats?"

Dr. Seuss

Okay, so Dr. Seuss didn't really say that, but he could have with all of the confusion about the role of fat in the modern diet. This is partially because of the mixed medical data around saturated fats and polyunsaturated fats, the relatively new support for Omega-3 fats, and the recent retreat from trans fats (also known as hydrogenated fats). Diets high in fat are also high in calories and contribute to obesity, which in turn is associated with an increased risk of cancer at several sites. Although all types of fats have similar numbers of calories, there are certain types, such as saturated fats, that may have a greater effect on increasing cancer risk. Current evidence suggests that it might be the type of fat in the diet rather than the total amount of fat that is most important to consider.

Dr. William Sears, a real doctor, has a very good way of describing fats. He believes that the low fat craze has caused people to avoid fats that they should actually eat. Dr. Sears says that people should follow a *right fat* diet, not a *low fat* diet. He believes that people should eat and enjoy monounsaturated and Omega-3 fats, limit animal fats (saturated fat), and avoid man-made fats (trans fats/hydrogenated fats).

Monounsaturated fat is a healthy fat to consume. It is a natural fat occurring in olive oil, canola oil, avocadoes, almonds, peanuts, unprocessed peanut butter, cashews and pecans. Unlike other fats, monounsaturated fat does not increase cholesterol. In fact, monounsaturated fat actually lowers bad cholesterol without lowering good cholesterol. It is recommended that you enjoy monounsaturated fat in substitution for other fats in your diet.

Omega-3 fat is also a healthy fat to consume. It appears to reduce inflammation in joints, reduce the risk of heart disease and may help reduce blood pressure levels. Omega-3 fat is a natural fat found in oily cold water fish (salmon, sardines, mackerel, herring, etc.) flax seeds, pumpkin seeds, walnuts, and eggs from chickens that have been fed Omega-3 fat. It is also recommended that you enjoy Omega-3 fat in substitution for other fats in your diet. Important Note: Omega-3 fat can be destroyed by heat and light. To preserve their healthful benefits, avoid overcooking fish and don't heat flax seed oil or expose it to light.

For years we have heard that saturated fats lead to cancer and heart disease, but there is some recent data to the contrary. Saturated fat does raise bad cholesterol (LDL), but it also raises good cholesterol (HDL). Saturated fat is found in beef, pork, poultry, dairy products like butter, cheese, milk and cream, coconut oil and palm oil. In my opinion, there is far more evidence to suggest that saturated fat is unhealthy, particularly in light of the industrial toxins stored in the fat of conventionally raised livestock, so I generally recommend that you limit your consumption of saturated fat.

Polyunsaturated fat was, in the 1960's and 1970's, thought to be a safe alternative to saturated fat. However, we have discovered that it is chemically unstable. It reacts with oxygen and forms carcinogenic compounds. Polyunsaturated fat can easily oxidize and begin forming free radicals in the body. Polyunsaturated fats can be found in mayonnaise, salad dressing, safflower oil, sunflower oil, corn oil and some vegetable oils. It is recommended that you avoid polyunsaturated fat.

Trans fat, also called trans fatty acid, hydrogenated fat or hydrogenated oil, should be eliminated from your diet altogether. Trans fat is a man-made fat created by superheating liquid unsaturated fat and injecting hydrogen into it to make it solid at room temperature. Studies show that trans fat increases bad cholesterol (LDL) and decreases good cholesterol (HDL) and trans fats have been linked to an increased risk of cancer and heart disease. Trans fat has been shown to decrease the body's ability to produce natural substances that regulate many of the body's functions and it may even interfere with the ability of the cells of the body to metabolize the fats that are good for you. Trans fats can be found in margarine, most processed peanut butter, pastries, packaged snacks, crackers, cookies, cereal and vegetable shortening. In addition, many foods served at restaurants contain trans fat, especially fried foods like French fries. Restaurants typically do not disclose trans fat content and it is used in many, many foods that you eat out. Trans fats/hydrogenated fats should be avoided.

Fortunately, on January 1, 2006, the Food & Drug Administration made changes to food labeling laws required the listing of trans fat on food labels. However, to be sure that there are actually no trans fats in the foods you buy at the store, you will have to go past the "0 g of trans fat" advertisement on the front of the package and read the ingredient list to ensure that no hydrogenated oils are listed. Just because the package says "0g of trans fat" does not mean that the product you are buying is actually free of trans fat. The FDA allows food manufacturers to list 0g of trans fat if there is less than .5g of trans fat per serving.

This is interesting, so let me explain. Food manufacturers with products based on cheap trans fats don't actually have to remove the unhealthy trans fat from their products. All they actually have to do to meet the FDA requirements (and to fool the consumer) is to decrease their serving size on the label until there is less than .5g of trans fat per serving. For example, many cereals advertise "0 g of trans fat" on the front of the cereal box, but a closer examination reveals hydrogenated fats in the ingredient list. Mores study of the cereal box label reveals that the cereal manufacturers list their serving sizes at between ½ cup and ¾ cup (about a handful), which is an amount far smaller than the serving that the average person eats. So, the cereal manufacturers kept the known toxic ingredient in their products, but adjusted the serving size until the "trans fat per serving" was below the FDA limit. Whatever generates a profit, right guys?

This may be the best example I know of the profit motive's absolute disregard for human health. As you have read above, trans fat is scientifically proven to be absolutely toxic to the human body, but it is a cheap ingredient with properties that are hard to duplicate inexpensively. So, food manufacturers lobbied the FDA to include a loophole in its labeling law on trans fat so that they could continue to use it but fool consumers into believing that they were protecting their families from the toxic stuff. Many shoppers seek out products that advertise "0 g of trans fat" because they have heard that trans fat is unhealthy. In reality, they are feeding their families the same unhealthy product formulation as before, but the manufacturer used a mathematical trick to fool them into believing that they were making a healthier choice! Unbelievable! Alright, I am climbing down off of my soap box (for now).

In summary, you should eat 30 or fewer grams of fat per day, with more of it in the form of monounsaturated fat and Omega-3 fat. You should limit the amount of saturated animal fat that you eat, avoid polyunsaturated fats like vegetable oil, and do your absolute best to eliminate foods that contain trans fats (at stores and restaurants).

If you are as confused as Dr. Seuss, below is a table that might help you sort out the confusion around fat and oils.

Type of Fat	Often Found In	Guidance
Monounsaturated Fat	Olive oil, canola oil, avocadoes, almonds, peanuts, unprocessed peanut butter, cashews, pecans	Enjoy
Omega-3 Fats	Oily cold water fish (salmon, sardines, mackerel, herring) flax seeds, pumpkin seeds, walnuts, and eggs from chickens that have been fed Omega-3 fat	Include
Saturated Fat	Beef, pork, poultry, dairy products like butter, cheese, milk & cream, coconut and palm oils	Limit
Polyunsaturated Fat	Vegetable oil, sesame oil, sunflower oil, safflower oil, corn oil, cottonseed oil, most mayonnaise, many salad dressings	Avoid
Trans Fat/ Hydrogenated Fat	Margarine, vegetable shortening, some salad dressings, many processed and packaged foods like cookies, crackers, chips, pastries, doughnuts, processed peanut butter, fried foods, fast food, some salad dressings, some bagels, some soups	Eliminate

Do Supplements Make a Difference in Health or Not?
There are 13 known vitamins and 22 known essential minerals, but they cannot be manufactured by the human body, so we get these from the food we consume and, increasingly, from nutritional supplements. In 2005, nearly $21 billion worth of vitamin and nutrition supplements were sold according to the *Nutrition Business Journal*. It is believed that nearly half the population of the U.S. takes one or more supplement.

Vitamin and mineral supplements are cheap and easy to get, giving people the quick gratification that they've taken a small step towards protecting their well-being. There is a commonly held belief that the consumption of vitamin and mineral supplements can make up for the lack of quality nutrients in the food you eat (no doubt a result of effective marketing). However, a multivitamin is not an insurance policy against disease or a guarantee of longevity. In fact, there is limited clinical data on the benefits that supplements offer to healthy adults.

Many supplements contain nothing more than inert laboratory chemicals that scientists argue are not processed by the body in the same way as the food-based vitamins that they are replacing. In addition, consuming the *combinations* of vitamins and minerals found *only* in foods is believed to be as important in meeting nutritional needs as getting the recommended daily allowances of individual vitamins and minerals. In other words, laboratory-developed vitamin and mineral supplements cannot compete with the valuable combinations of nutrients provided by nature.

A sales coach and author friend of mine, Rick Page, tells a great selling story about a certain brand of septic tank cleaner. He uses this product to describe how people will buy anything that they *believe* in. He illustrates this by describing how consumers buy this septic tank cleaner once per month, pour it into the toilet and, quite literally, flush it down the drain with no immediate effect. However, consumers walk away from the toilet with great peace of mind because they *believe* that they are preventing a really awful septic backup. In a way, this is a little bit like taking vitamins and minerals. You buy these bottles of pills, pop them in your mouth and notice no immediate effects until alarmingly yellow urine leaves your body for the sewer, but you have peace of mind because you *believe* that you have done something good for your health. Vitamins and minerals may, in fact, be little more than just another substance for the body to excrete, at least for a healthy adult. (Now before you religious-vitamin-takers-who-thought-you-liked-me dismiss me as an enemy of the soon-to-be-discovered truth, read on.)

Whole, organic foods (ones that have not been modified by man from their original state) have vitamins and minerals that are in natural harmony with one another. That is, each vitamin or mineral in a whole, organic food exists in its original chemical form and in its natural proportion to the other elements in the food. Scientists have not yet discovered or identified all of the nutrients in whole foods and they have also not determined how all of the nutrients interplay with one another and the effect of the interplay on the body. Therefore, man cannot manufacture a vitamin or mineral supplement that can mimic nature. As a result, you cannot expect vitamin and mineral supplements to provide your body with the nutrition it needs to maintain its harmony. You must get your primary nutrition from whole, organic foods.

However, having said all of that, there are a large number of people in modern societies falling short of their recommended daily allowances of vitamins and minerals. The processing, storage and cooking that strips vitamins and minerals from food, the modern fast-food diet consumed by so many, and the reduced minerals available in the soil results in an over-fed, under-nourished population. If you do not consume a broad array of the recommended servings of fruits, vegetables, grains, beans, low fat dairy, lean meats, etc., then you probably could benefit form a vitamin and mineral supplement. Remember, the body will go on reproducing the cells that it needs to survive, but if it does not have the basic nutrients it needs, the cells will be "defective," fewer in number and more easily damaged or destroyed. If this situation becomes chronic, it can, and probably will, lead to many health problems including degenerative disease.

Among the limited data available on the benefits of vitamins and minerals, there are some encouraging nuggets:

- Solid evidence exists that the folate in a multivitamin benefits women and their fetuses during pregnancy.
- Evidence suggests a regular multivitamin may offer some benefit to subgroups of patients who have chronic conditions.
- In a clinical trial, men who took vitamin E (50 mg/day) had a lower risk of prostate cancer compared with men who took a placebo.
- Harvard researchers reported that "long-term use of multivitamins may substantially reduce the risk for colon cancer."
- Harvard researchers found that taking a multivitamin delayed the progression of HIV.
- Vitamin and mineral supplements have been shown to reduce the risk of stomach cancer in studies of malnourished people in China and South America.

- Researchers found that type 2 diabetes patients who took a daily multivitamin had a significantly lower rate of infection compared with those who took a placebo.

If you do take a vitamin and mineral supplement, it is recommended that you take a balanced multivitamin/mineral supplement containing no more than 100% of the "Daily Value" of most nutrients to ensure that you are not taking too much of any single nutrient because high doses of some nutrients can have harmful effects. The supplement industry is a multi-billion dollar industry that encourages people to buy individual vitamins and minerals and, essentially, become their own pharmacist. In many cases, it is not known which compounds or combination of compounds is most beneficial to our health. So, introducing nutrients in a piecemeal fashion is an uncertain route to take when trying to improve your overall nutrition. While it is true that no one ever died from an overdose of beta carotene because he ate too many carrots or an overdose of vitamin C because he ate too many oranges, the same cannot be said for vitamin and mineral pills. Don't be fooled into thinking that you are better safe than sorry and take vitamins and minerals to excess. We do know that too much of a chemical or too little of a chemical can be a bad thing in our bodies. Just like we shouldn't let doctors partner with drug companies to run chemical experiments on our bodies, we shouldn't partner with supplement companies to do this either.

It is also important, in my opinion, that you take a vitamin or mineral supplement that is food-based. That is, the vitamins and minerals contained in the pill should be from food sources, not laboratory sources. Look for the words "food-based" on the label. And, because it is not what is in the bottle but what gets into your bloodstream that matters, I recommend that you take half the recommended daily allowance twice per day as opposed to taking it all at once. If supplements do not get into the bloodstream, they pass right through body and exit in a bright yellow stream of 'sewer nutrition.'

There is another category of "supplement" that I think is worth mentioning: concentrated fruit and vegetable supplements. This type of supplement is different from both laboratory-derived and "food-based" vitamin and mineral supplements. These supplements contain the dried juice of whole fruits and vegetables in a pill. I like this type of supplement because it delivers whole foods in concentrated form and is a convenient way to increase variety of phytonutrients in your diet. There are several brands available, but I like the Juice Plus brand because it has the dried juice of pure, organic fruits and vegetables in a pill.

In summary, supplements are not intended to replace a healthy diet. They are called "supplements" because they are intended to fill gaps in a healthy diet – and a healthy diet is the cornerstone of a healthy body.

Reading Food Labels

If you want to be healthy, it is critical that you know what you are putting in your body. Therefore, you need to make a habit of reading food labels and you need to know what to look for. Food labels follow an FDA standard and below is a quick primer on the things you need to know.

Serving size is the first measure on the label. Food manufacturers choose their serving sizes based on what will look good in the "Amount Per Serving" section listed below it, not based on the serving size that the typical person will eat (marketing never sleeps). The first thing you should do when you look at a food label is try to envision the amount of this food that you will actually eat and compare that to the serving size. Often times, you will eat two to three times the serving size in one sitting. If this is the case, then all of the items listed in the Amount Per Serving section on the label should be multiplied by this factor in order to get an accurate reading of how much of each item you will be eating per true serving.

Nutrition Facts

Serving Size ½ cup (114g)
Servings Per Container 4

Amount Per Serving

Calories 90   Calories from Fat 30

	% Daily Value*
Total Fat 3g	5%
Saturated Fat 0g	0%
Cholesterol 0mg	0%
Sodium 300mg	13%
Total Carbohydrate 13g	4%
Dietary Fiber 3g	12%
Sugars 3g	
Protein 3g	

Vitamin A	80%	•	Vitamin C	80%
Calcium	4%	•	Iron	4%

* Percent Daily Values are based on a 2,000 calorie diet. Your daily values may be higher or lower depending on your calorie needs:

	Calories	2,000	2,500
Total Fat	Less than	65g	80g
Sat Fat	Less than	20g	25g
Cholesterol	Less than	300mg	300mg
Sodium	Less than	2,400mg	2,400mg
Total Carbohydrate		300g	375g
Fiber		25g	30g

Calories per gram:
Fat 9   •   Carbohydrate 4   •   Protein 4

Total fat, saturated fat, trans fat, cholesterol and sodium are the first nutrients listed on a food's label. These are nutrients that the FDA believes that Americans generally eat in adequate amounts. They are listed in grams and are shown in comparison to the percentage daily value of a 2,000 calorie diet (except for trans fat, which has no daily value). Guidelines recommend the intake of these be as low as possible.

Earlier in this chapter, there is a detailed discussion on fat that should help you make more informed decisions when reading food labels. However, sodium has not yet been addressed. Sodium is salt and we Westerners eat far too much of it. The average person in America consumes between 10 and 20 grams of salt per day. Excessive use of salt and being overweight are the two leading causes of high blood pressure in roughly 60 million Americans. The American Lung Association recommends eating less than 2,400 milligrams of salt per day (about one tablespoon).

I also recommend that you pay close attention to the listing of sugar on food labels. The amount of "sugars" is listed under Total Carbohydrates in grams. Westerners also eat far too much sugar. The average American consumes over 150 pounds of sugar each year and nearly 11,000 pounds of sugar in his or her lifetime. That is nearly the weight of two Chevrolet Suburbans! I discuss the perils of eating too much sugar in an upcoming chapter, but suffice it to say that you need to eat a lot less of the stuff.

Finally, the FDA reports that most Americans don't eat enough fiber, vitamins A and C, calcium, and iron, so these nutrients are also listed on food labels. They are shown primarily by percentage daily value, but dietary fiber is also shown in grams. In addition, food labels list the percent daily values on which its percentages are based toward the bottom for reference.

Building Your Diet around Nature's Harvest
Many people cannot imagine themselves changing their eating habits because they believe that it would be too difficult to maintain the habit of healthy eating. In Part III of this book, I have included a foolproof system for adopting habits that can be customized to meet your specific circumstances. This system was created to help you more easily adopt the eight habits of healthy people.

That said, however, it is important that you know that this program is not all or nothing. Every meal doesn't have to meet all the guidelines that I have laid out. You need to cheat now and again so that the program doesn't feel so rigorous that you fall off the wagon completely. For example, I tend to cheat on one meal per week, typically lunch on Friday. What is important is that you apply the guidelines to your overall eating pattern so that the vast majority of the food you eat comes from nature's harvest.

Adopting a diet based on nature's harvest is one of the key cornerstones to long-term health. The alternative modern diet is simply ill-suited for our genetic composition. Our development has not kept pace with advances in agriculture and food processing resulting in a plague of health problems for modern man. Coronary heart disease, diabetes, cancer, osteoporosis, obesity and psychological dysfunction have all been scientifically linked to a diet too high in refined foods.

In plain language, base your diet on fruits, vegetables, grains, lean meats, beans, nuts and seeds, little processed food, and limited sugar. That's about as simple as I can make it. If you follow these simple guidelines, you will benefit from nearly all that can be achieved through nutrition.

In a Nutshell: The Live on Nature's Harvest Rules
1. To properly nourish your body, half or more of your food should be fresh, raw, living food.
2. In general, the thing to remember about fruits and vegetables is that you simply cannot eat too many. Also remember that variety may be as important as quantity.
3. Inspect product labels to ensure that you are getting whole grain products. Whole grains have considerably more fiber and nutrients than refined (or processed) grains.
4. Eat more nuts, beans and seeds. Analyses show that people who eat these foods regularly consume more vitamins and minerals and tend to outlive individuals who don't.
5. Strictly limit fatty cuts of meat, saturated fat, polyunsaturated fat (vegetable oil) and hydrogenated fat (margarine, shortening). Instead try to buy lean cuts of meat and low fat dairy products (both organic if you can afford it) and wild, cold water fish.

A Word about the 8 Habits of Healthy People

If you are beginning to worry about the challenge of adopting these habits, don't. There is an activity in Part III of this book that will help you prioritize the habits that you need to adopt and a simple approach to help you adopt them and make them a routine part of your life. In addition, there is an entire website (www.habitsofhealth.com) devoted to helping you adopt The 8 Habits of Healthy People with an abundance of great resources.

Chapter 6

Drink from the Fountain of Health

Water is the only drink for a wise man.
Henry David Thoreau

Certainly, you have heard the expression, *you are what you eat*. We know that this is a euphemism because none of us is really a tomato or a hamburger. However, when it comes to what you drink, it is entirely accurate to say that *you are what you drink*. The human body is made up of approximately 66% water. Our muscles and brains are over 75% water, our blood is approximately 82% water, our bones are approximately 25% water, and our liver is almost 96% water. Nearly everything that happens inside of our bodies - including digestion, nutrient distribution, energy production and detoxification - happens with water. Without a sufficient intake of water, your cells can not carry nutrients to your body's vital organs or effectively dispose of waste. Over time, a deficiency of water *directly* results in a variety of degenerating conditions including headaches, back pain, hypertension, arthritis and asthma. As you will read, a deficiency of water in the body can also *indirectly* contribute to more serious chronic conditions such as cancer.

Water, Water Everywhere, but Not a Drop to Drink
The same amount of water that exists on earth today existed millions of years ago. Our planet continuously recycles its finite supply of water. With the understanding that water is vital to nearly every function in our body, it is easy to grasp the importance of having plenty of pure, clean water. It's also important to realize that it is not just important to have clean drinking water. We have to have clean cooking water and clean water as the primary ingredient of our other drinks – juices, coffee, tea, etc. In addition, we also need clean bathing water because the skin, the body's largest organ, absorbs the elements in water and we inhale the steam of a hot shower. Once we realize that everything that goes down the drain, on our lawns, on farm fields, or into the environment eventually winds up in our water supply, we begin to see just how vulnerable this planet's water really is.

While the standard use in our society of over 80,000 different synthetic chemicals has improved convenience and productivity, it has also come at a tremendous price: drastic increases in chemical pollution. Our use of man-made chemicals has become so extreme that we can now find traces of these chemicals in virtually every public water supply around the world. Over five hundred billion pounds of synthetic chemicals are produced every year. As those chemicals are used in manufacturing, transportation, energy production, agriculture and simple daily life, an alarmingly large amount winds up in our lakes, rivers, streams and ground water.

Pesticides are a grand example. Every year in the United States, over two billion pounds of pesticides, herbicides and fungicides (collectively known as pesticides) are spread onto fields of commercial crops and home lawns and gardens. That is nearly seven pounds of pesticides per year for every man, woman and child living in America. Rains wash a sizeable portion of those chemicals right into the drinking water supply.

A 1998 study of 29 major U.S. cities by the Environmental Working Group found that all 29 cities had traces of at least one weed killer in the drinking water. The same group found that Americans in 245 communities are exposed to levels of carcinogenic herbicides in drinking water that exceed the EPA's benchmark of acceptable cancer risk. One sample from a suburb of Cincinnati contained ten different herbicides, and samples from five other towns in Ohio and Illinois contained at least six herbicides. If only 5% of the pesticides applied every year in the U.S. were to wash into the drinking water supply, it could result in sixty million pounds of pesticides going into our bodies every year (assuming 40% of our water supply is used for non-consumption activities such as washing dishes and clothes, flushing toilets and watering lawns). While that only amounts to about $1/5^{th}$ of a pound of pesticide per American per year, the average fifty-year old would have consumed ten pounds of pesticides in his or her lifetime.

Why does this matter? Along with other toxic chemicals, pesticides contain neurotoxins, chemicals that attack the nervous systems of insects. If you ingest $1/5^{th}$ of a pound of neurotoxins every year for 30, 40 or 50 years (consuming 6 pounds, 8 pounds or 10 pounds of neurotoxins respectively), how bad will that be for your nervous system? Could that have something to do with the increases in neurological disorders and diseases like Lou Gehrig's disease, Parkinson's disease, dementia, multiple sclerosis, Huntington's disease, brain cancer, cerebral palsy, autism and Alzheimer's? Could it be contributing to the increased incidence of migraine headaches, sleep disorders, attention deficit disorders, memory loss, hyperactivity and depression? Scientists will tell you that there is not enough evidence to meet their standard of scientific proof. I say that there is too much evidence to sit idle and wait for science to mature enough to provide us with scientific proof.

There are also contaminants like chlorine and lead in our drinking water supplies that do not get there as a result of accidental chemical runoff. The addition of chlorine to our water began in the late 1800s to fight water-borne diseases such as typhoid and cholera, and for the most part, this remains the standard today. No one will argue that chlorine serves an important purpose. However, we don't use chlorine because it's the safest or even the most effective means of disinfection. We use it because it is the cheapest. In spite of all our technological advances, we essentially still pour bleach into our water prior to consumption.

There is a lot of well-founded concern about chlorine. In particular, during the chlorination process itself, chlorine combines with decaying vegetation to form potent cancer causing trihalomethanes (THM's). These chlorine by-products trigger the production of free radicals in the body, causing cell damage, and are highly carcinogenic. According to the U.S. Council of Environmental Quality, "Cancer risk among people using chlorinated water is as much as 93% higher than among those whose water does not contain chlorine." Chlorine is also suspected to contribute to hardening of the arteries, the primary cause of heart disease.

Next to chlorine, lead is the most common contaminant found in tap water. Lead in drinking water usually originates between the water main at the curb and the household faucet, so treatment from a central point does not help. The EPA estimates that 98% of all homes have pipes, fixtures or solder joints in the household plumbing that can leach some level of lead into the tap water. Homes built before 1986 are more likely to have lead pipes, fixtures and solder. However, new homes are at risk too: modern fixtures labeled "lead-free" can contain 8% to 15% lead, which can leach into water, especially hot water (sounds a little like the "trans-fat free" labeling requirement. Whose interest does our government represent anyway?)

Lead exposure is cumulative and long-lasting in humans. This toxic metal gets stored by the body, primarily in bones and teeth. It has been determined that there is no safe level for lead in drinking water, especially for small children (the EPA Maximum Contaminant Level Goal is 0 parts per billion). Even very low levels of lead can cause irreversible damage to children such as reduced IQs, learning disabilities and behavioral problems. In adults, lead in drinking water causes high blood pressure, reduces hemoglobin production, and interferes with normal calcium metabolism. Unfortunately, lead found in drinking water often exceeds the EPA's legal limit of 15 parts per billion and it is estimated that lead in drinking water contributes to 500,000 cases of learning disorders in children and 560,000 cases of hypertension in adults every year in the U.S.

Water (Mis) Treatment
The earth's natural filtration process is not effective at removing toxic chemicals and unfortunately, neither is municipal water treatment. Most of us believe that the water that is supplied to our homes is clean and highly filtered. If you think that your water utility effectively cleans your drinking water before you drink it, consider this: caffeine, nicotine, antibiotics and many prescription drugs are now being detected at the point of consumption in many water systems around the world. How do you think those got into your drinking water? It is not a very pleasant thought, but it is estimated that about 10% of the water we drink has been used before (and I think you know what I mean by *used*). If these things are in our drinking water, they were certainly there when the water got to the treatment plant, but the treatment facilities were unable to effectively clean them out of the water. Our municipal water treatment facilities do not remove synthetic chemicals and typically consist only of sand bed filtration and disinfection, much like a standard swimming pool filter. For the most part, today's water treatment facilities are much the same as they were at the turn of the century.

On October 1, 1999, a new federal law went into effect that requires water utilities to send each customer a detailed report showing what is in their water, appropriately called "The Right to Know Amendment." These reports detail the level of certain contaminants in the drinking water supply and identify the Environmental Protection Agency's MCLG (Maximum Contaminant Level Goal) and MCL (Maximum Contaminant Level) for each contaminant. The MCLG is the level at which the

Environmental Protection Agency has determined that unacceptable health risks may occur. The MCL is the level at which the Environmental Protection Agency requires corrective action and can impose penalties. Notice that the MCLG is always at or below the MCL. Understand this point: The government does not require corrective action when the contaminant level reaches the MCLG (where unacceptable health risks may occur), only when contaminant levels reach the MCL. So, it is important to understand that a "superior" water system only means that it complies with EPA minimum water quality standards, not that it doesn't contain unhealthy levels of contaminants.

And these reports are in no way complete. Of the over 80,000 toxic chemicals used in our society, the EPA has only set drinking water standards for 90 (~1%) and the water utilities are only required to test for those 90 contaminants. According to a report entitled Troubled Waters on Tap, "over 2100 contaminants have been detected in U. S. drinking water since 1974 with 190 known or suspected to cause adverse health effects at certain concentration levels. In total, 97 carcinogens and suspected carcinogens, 82 mutagens and suspected mutagens, 28 acute and chronic toxic contaminants and 23 tumor promoters have been detected in U. S. drinking water since 1974."

And the FDA only requires that water utilities test for 90 contaminants? In addition, the Maximum Contaminant Levels (MCL's) for the 90 that water utilities are required to test for are set based on consumption of one specific chemical by a healthy 175 pound adult. No consideration is given to the effects on infants, children, pregnant women and their fetuses, the elderly, or the chronically ill. Infants and children are at particular risk because they drink more than two and a half times as much water as adults as a proportion of their body weight. In addition, there is no testing on the effects of two or more contaminants when combined, which some studies show are magnified by as much as 1,000 times.

Recently, I received my "Right to Know" report from my municipal water company along with my semi-monthly bill. I have to admit, in spite of the fact that I have become a student of the effect of our toxic world on human health, I have never really read the annually produced report on my municipal water quality. Since I drink bottled and purified water and shower in filtered water, I guess I never really paid attention. To my great shock, upon reading the report, I learned that my municipal water is supplied by none other than the Chattahoochee River. I'll admit, in retrospect, I'm not sure where else the water would have come from given that the river is the only major source of water near my home north of Atlanta, Georgia. However, my shock came from the knowledge that the Chattahoochee River is so polluted that it is widely known that you *cannot* eat the fish caught there due to PCB contamination (polychlorinated biphenyl), but my family, and the families all around me, were suppose to drink this stuff?

The following passage appeared in a report produced by the Georgia Department of Natural Resources in 2003 regarding PCB levels found in fish in the Chattahoochee River:

"PCBs are a group of synthetic organic chemicals that contain 209 possible individual chlorinated biphenyl compounds... Although banned in the United States from further production in 1979, PCBs are distributed widely in the environment because of their persistence and widespread use... PCB exposure is associated with a wide array of adverse health effects in experimental animals. Experimental animal studies have shown toxic effects to the liver, gastrointestinal system, blood, skin, endocrine system, immune system, nervous system, and reproductive system. In addition, developmental effects and liver cancer have been reported. Skin rashes and a severe form of acne have been documented in humans; however, other effects of PCB exposure in humans are not well understood. The EPA has classified PCBs as probable human carcinogens (Group B2)."

I am not an expert on water quality or water treatment, but if the state Department of Natural Resources strictly limits the number of fish that you should eat out of a body of water because of carcinogenic contamination, and the water treatment facilities are unable to filter out that carcinogenic contamination, why the $%@!# are my neighbors and I allowed to drink an unlimited supply of it out of the tap without warning? Am I supposed to feel safe because they filter out the sediment and pour chlorine into it before they send it through galvanized pipes into my house? Am I the only one who noticed this?

After the 9/11 attack that left people afraid to fly, the CEO of one of the major airlines flew aboard one of his planes in a publicity stunt to demonstrate that there was nothing to fear. I wonder if the people that work at the EPA would be willing to commit to drinking only tap water for a year. Carol Browner, the current (and longest serving) Chief Administrator of the U.S. Environmental Protection Agency said recently, "The way we guarantee safe drinking water is broken and needs to be fixed." Her predecessor, William Reilly, said, "Drinking water in the U.S. is among the top four public health risks posed by environmental problems." My guess is that they wouldn't accept my challenge, and you shouldn't either.

I strongly recommend that you only drink and use purified water or spring water from a trusted source. Our municipal water supply is polluted and getting worse every day. Later in this chapter, I provide more specific recommendations.

Drink Up
After learning more about our increasingly polluted water supply, you could easily come away with the impression that drinking water is bad for your health. To the contrary, drinking plenty of *clean, pure* water is one of the most important things you can do to improve and maintain your health. As was discussed at the outset of this chapter, the human body is two-thirds water and every major function in the human body depends on an adequate supply. You, quite literally, are what you drink.

For years, we have been told that we should drink a minimum of eight 8 ounce glasses of water each day (for a total of 64 ounces). The world we live in today is much different than it was 70 years ago when this recommendation was first made in medical journals. We are exposed to a multitude of toxic chemicals and environmental pollutants that didn't even exist prior to the 1960's. The resulting accumulation of chemical toxins requires an increased intake of clean water to compensate for the increased physiological stress.

Today, the average man needs to consume three quarts of water every day and the average woman needs to consume two quarts (1 quart = 32 ounces = ~ two 16

How much clean water do you need?

$$\text{Min. Water Need/ Day (ounces)} = \frac{\text{Body Weight}}{2}$$

ounce bottles of water). However, as my mother would say, "None of us is average." So, here is a good rule of thumb to determine your individual water needs: divide your body weight by two to get the *minimum* number of ounces of water that you need to consume every day. For example, a 155 pound person would need to consume at least 78 ounces of clean, pure water every single day in order to maintain his health. To give that number some context, a 155 pound person would need to drink five, 16 ounce bottles of water per day to reach the *minimum* recommendation.

If you are a person who does not drink much water today, don't be scared away by the thought of drinking this much water every day. Before I became sick and changed my habits, I never drank water. I couldn't stand drinking it. I used to say, "Water is for swimming, showering and sh_tting." To me, it had no taste and even made me nauseas.

Today, with the exception of organic coffee and the occasional fruit smoothie, water is all I ever drink. I found that once I started drinking more water, I craved it. As my sensory addiction to the manufactured taste of soft drinks wore off, I really began to enjoy the refreshment that only clean, pure water can provide. Now that drinking water is a routine, I easily drink 90 ounces of water every day (I weigh 175 pounds). In fact, today, I feel like something is missing – like I have forgotten something – if I do not have water within arm's reach.

Fortunately, drinking H2O is not the only source of water for your body. If you build your diet around nature's harvest as the previous chapter recommends, you will also get a lot of water in the foods you eat. Fruits and vegetables, for example, are typically more than 60% water. Like fruits and vegetables, fruit and vegetable juices contain a lot of water and can help you meet your daily consumption target, too. Unfortunately for you coffee and soda drinkers, you cannot count the water contained in caffeinated or carbonated beverages because these drinks often have a diuretic effect.

However you get it, you need to try to spread your clean water consumption out throughout the day. This gives your cells, tissues and organs a constant supply of clean water. Oh, and by the way, it will also help to control your appetite.

There is a twist to this, however. While you should spread your water consumption throughout the day, you should actually avoid drinking very much at meal time. Yes, you read that correctly. Drink more water, but reduce your consumption of liquid, especially cold liquid, when you eat. This is because fluids, which are digested before solid foods, can carry away the enzymes needed for digestion and cold fluids can cool down the stomach which needs heat to aid digestion. I know it is culturally weird (in the same way that not having debt is), but it does make a difference in your nutrition. Why wash away all the nutrients you have worked so hard to consume? (To avoid the raised eyebrows when you turn down a drink with a meal, simply ask for water and let it sit next to your plate. No one will notice when you don't drink it.)

Drinking From the Fountain of Health
Getting plenty of clean, pure water is critical to your health and it needn't be a burden. Below are six steps to easily turn your water supply into a fountain of health.

Know what you get out of the tap. Because you really can't avoid the using the water in your home, you should make the effort to remain informed about your municipal supply. Your water suppliers can tell you the lakes, rivers, and groundwater sources from which your water comes. You can also ask for or search the Internet for copies of your public water system's monitoring results for both regulated and unregulated contaminants in the water. In addition, you can find copies of any public notices they have issued regarding violations over the past few years.

Purchase point-of-use water filters for your home that are effective against the known risks in your water supply. With point-of-use filtration of your drinking, bathing and cooking water, you can significantly reduce the toxic chemicals entering your body. Buy one unit for the kitchen to take the risks of many pollutants and chemicals out of your drinking and cooking water and buy shower filters for your high-use showers (substantial amounts of chlorine can enter the body through inhaled steam in hot showers).

The most effective means of filtering water include some combination of two or more of the following: reverse osmosis, sub-micron filtration, activated charcoal filtration, deionization and ion exchange filtration. Reverse osmosis and submicron filtration pull water through a membrane, trapping small particles in the water behind the membrane. A charcoal filter pulls water through a charcoal interface and particles in the water get trapped by the binding properties of charcoal. Deionozation and ion exchange filtration trap impurities by attracting their charged particles, removing them from the water. Because different purification methods trap different kinds of impurities, it is important to have a water filter that utilizes multiple filtration methods (which most filters built in to your refrigerator don't have).

Please note that filtration systems needn't be expensive. An entire home can be well equipped for less than $500. Choose carefully, however, as the water filtration business is largely unregulated. Many companies use bold marketing language and make unsubstantiated claims. Choose reputable brands and look for things like *Consumer Reports* reviews and certifications by an independent testing organization such as NSF International before choosing a model. Also, be sure to replace the filters at the manufacturer's recommended intervals or you can actually cause your water to become *more* polluted!

I use an inexpensive, yet highly effective, set of filters in my home from Sun Water Systems (www.aquasauna.com).

Drink purified bottled water. For water on the go, do some research on bottled water brands to learn about the quality of the water behind the label. Bottled water has historically had lower EPA standards than municipally supplied water so all bottled water is not created equal. Also, spring water can be contaminated with many of the same run-off chemicals as our streams, rivers and lakes. So, if you are not careful about the bottled water you buy, you might be getting dirtier water than you could get out of the tap and paying five times as much for it. I recommend that you buy *purified* bottled water that has been filtered using a combination of the methods mentioned above.

If you don't have easy access to bottled water on the go or if it doesn't fit your budget, purchase a water pitcher or sports bottle with a charcoal filter and keep it with you. These are also great to take with you when you travel to places where you can't guarantee access to affordable clean water.

Do not drink tap water (or fountain drinks like soda, tea or lemonade as they are made with tap water) at a restaurant. Order bottled water and do not take ice with it (most ice is not filtered). Or, don't drink anything. Many nutritionist recommend not drinking much if anything within two hours of a meal to aid in digestion.

Get into a watering routine. I always drink bottled water or a tall glass of filtered water when I exercise in the morning and again at bed time. These two routines have become so habitual that I don't even have to think about them any more. I feel that something is missing if I don't have my water during my workout or at my bedside. With these two out of the way, I only need to drink three more during the day, and I do that by "preloading."

Preload your drinking water. As described above, I get two of my "servings" of water from my morning and nighttime routines. So, to reach my minimum water consumption goal on a daily basis, I need to drink three or more servings of water at some time during the day. During a busy day, it is hard to remember to do this, especially since I don't drink with meals. So, I have developed the habit of "preloading" my water at the beginning of the day by getting all of the water that I need to drink and putting it on the desk in front of me where I work. It serves as a reminder to me to be drinking water all day long because I don't want to have to chug it all down just before I leave my office at night!

In a Nutshell: The Drink from the Fountain of Health Rules
1. Drinking plenty of *clean, pure* water is one of the most important things you can do to improve and maintain your health. Divide your body weight by two to get the minimum number of ounces of water that you need to consume every day.
2. Only consume water from a source you know is clean. Purified and spring water are the best choices (in that order).
3. Spread your water consumption out throughout the day to give your body a constant supply.
4. Reduce your consumption of liquid, especially cold liquid, when you eat.

Chapter 7

Be In-Dependent

Everything in excess is opposed by nature.

Hippocrates

Here it is folks – the chapter on quitting _bad_ habits. You knew was it was in here somewhere. You knew that there were things that you were doing that were not good for you, but you just hoped, by some miracle of modern scientific discovery, you wouldn't have to stop doing them. But alas, this is not the case.

We have all heard the medical idiom that begins, "First, do no harm." This is how you should view your health. Imagine health as a liquid and imagine your body as a bucket that contains some of this health liquid. If you have a leaky bucket, with health leaking out of the bottom, no matter how much health liquid you put into the bucket, it can never stay full. Put very simply, it is impossible to stay healthy when you have harmful, bad habits. They drain your health.

Let me assure you that this is, I know, the hardest habit. Because _dependency_ is often the result of a craving of some stimulus, it is harder to stop a bad habit than it is to start a good one. Also, many of our bad habits are supported by our social lives. However, if you are a smoker, a sugar addict or cannot imagine life without a 12-pack of beer every weekend, don't stop here and give up. There is plenty of hope. No matter how compulsive your dependencies are, experience has shown that they can be overcome with a little will power and a good support system like the one provided in Part III of this book. Also remember that there are eight other habits in this book and they all contribute to your health. You can begin to improve your health by developing other habits of health while you wean yourself off of your bad habits. In other words, you can increase the health liquid going into your bucket while slowing down the amount leaking out the bottom, eventually stabilizing at full health.

All of that said, this book is about health and I do not want to shy away from the fact that the dependencies listed here are significant contributors to the Cumulative Effect on your body. Most of our compulsive dependencies are extremely debilitating to the body's immune system and contribute to the accumulation of toxins in the body. Below, I have listed the dependencies that have the most detrimental effect on human health. I have listed them in an order that considers two factors: the severity of impact on overall health and the frequency of the dependency. If a dependency is severe and common, it is towards the top. As either severity or frequency decreases, the item falls further down on the list. For example, a narcotics dependency is considered severely detrimental to overall health, but it is less common than sugar dependency so it falls further down on the list.

Tobacco
When evaluating bad habits, it would be impossible to start with anything other than tobacco. More than 85% of lung cancers result from tobacco smoking and because there are no reliable methods for the early detection of lung cancer, it is most often diagnosed in its advanced stages. As a result, most lung cancer patients die within two years of being diagnosed. If current trends continue, tobacco-related deaths will increase from about 4 million per year today to 10 million per year in 2030. Based on current statistics, smoking-related diseases will kill about 500 million of the 1.2 billion smokers alive today. In China alone, where two-thirds of the male population smokes, it is estimated that smoking will kill 100 million of the 300 million Chinese men ages 0 – 29.

If you smoke tobacco or use smokeless tobacco, you are suicidal, uninformed or thickheaded and you will probably die from diseases caused by tobacco. Volumes have been written on the many ways tobacco ruins your health and, unless you have been living in a hole (filled with Marlboros and Skoal), you hear a voice in your subconscious begging you to stop every time you light up a cigarette or put in a chew. There are plenty of programs to help you quit, but, like anything else, you have to want to quit. If you are a tobacco user and you are reading this book, you *do* want to quit.

If the health risks are not enough to cause you to re-think tobacco use, consider this: tobacco can affect your career and earning potential. Because tobacco use costs an estimated $158 billion in health care costs and lost productivity annually, employers are finding ways get rid of and avoid hiring tobacco users. In a story too ironic too be made up, Scotts Miracle-Gro, one of the world's largest distributors of lawn chemicals (harmful pesticides) has threatened to fire any employee who smokes after a deadline set in the Fall of 2006. They intend to randomly test employees and if caught, employees will be fired. Because it directly impacts profitability and because there are no laws that prevent employers from discriminating against tobacco users, I predict that tobacco users will have higher unemployment and earn 20% - 30% less than their peers in a decade.

Despite the staggering statistics and overwhelming public pressure against it, one in five American adults smokes. Although most tobacco users genuinely want to quit, addiction to tobacco is true drug dependence, comparable in severity to opiates, amphetamines and cocaine. However, it is possible to quit if you genuinely want to be healthy. In the year 2000, over 44 million adults in the United States were former smokers and nearly 49% of adults living in the U.S. that had ever smoked, had stopped. The key to success, experience is showing, is multiple approaches, repeated attempts and ongoing support in order to maintain abstinence.

When considering tobacco's affect on human health, it is important to understand that the diseases associated with using tobacco are, for the most part, manufactured into the product. According to a study presented to the American Thoracic Society Conference in 2006 (May 23 by Donald Tashkin, M.D., Professor of Medicine at UCLA), people who regularly smoke marijuana, even for extended periods of time, do not have an increased risk of cancer of the lungs, mouth, tongue, throat or esophagus. Marijuana has four times the amount of tar found in cigarettes and marijuana smokers tend to hold smoke in their lungs twice as long as tobacco smokers. Yet, there was no correlation found in the study between marijuana use, even long term marijuana use, and cancer risk.

My point in sharing this study is not to encourage you to dust off your bong. It is to illustrate that the act of *smoking* itself does not appear to cause cancer. In fact, studies of primitive cultures show that smoking naturally grown, unprocessed tobacco plants does not create the rate of disease that we see with processed tobacco consumption. As mentioned earlier, it has been found that the inhabitants of Kitava, an island off of the coast of Papua New Guinea, have an almost nonexistent rate of cardiac disease and stroke despite the fact that nearly 80% of the population smoke naturally grown tobacco.

Not unlike modern food manufacturing, tobacco production takes relatively benign natural plants and turns them into synthetic killers laced with degenerating toxins to make the product more addictive and more appealing. Over 2,000 chemicals are released every time a mass-produced cigarette is lit up. Tobacco use (unless you get your tobacco from Kitava) is the non-stop speed train to the cemetery. If you smoke or chew tobacco, you are committing suicide. Unless that is your intention, you have to stop.

Sugar
Are you surprised to see the sugar habit so high on the list (right after tobacco)? You shouldn't be. In the last twenty years, the average American has increased his annual sugar consumption from 26 pounds to over 150 pounds! It is estimated that Americans get nearly 25% of their caloric intake from sugar. At the current rate, the average American will eat 11,000 pounds of sugar in his or her lifetime.

Primarily because of the sensory pleasure derived from its appealing taste, sugar leads to addictive eating behavior more than any other food. I should know. I was a confirmed sugar addict. As a teenager, I would eat toast with gobs of jelly, honey or cinnamon sugar for breakfast, drink three or four Cherry Cokes or Dr Peppers during the day, and have a bowl of ice cream, a cup full of M&M's, or a candy bar after dinner. I grew up eating this way and I didn't know any better. Knowing what I know today, I am convinced that this is the primary reason that the Cumulative Effect was strong enough in my body to make me chronically ill.

Sugar, in the large quantities common to the standard American diet, creates a wide range of adverse reactions in the human body. Sugar can cause a significant rise in triglycerides, promote an elevation of harmful cholesterol (LDLs), increase the risk of coronary heart disease and hypertension, lead to elevated insulin levels, increase cancer risk, result in kidney damage, contribute to diabetes and hypoglycemia, cause free radical formation in the bloodstream, cause a deficiency in chromium and copper in the body, interfere with absorption of calcium and magnesium, contribute to osteoporosis, and lead to hyperactivity, anxiety, depression, concentration difficulties and hormonal imbalances. The most significant impact of sugar consumption, however, is its effect on the immune system. Sugar temporarily impairs the body's ability to produce antibodies to fight infection. Bad bacteria in the digestive tract thrive on high carbohydrate, high sugar foods and when you have a bacterial imbalance in your intestines, your immune system breaks down. With so much refined sugar in the "modern" diet, it is no surprise that we are prone to getting sick all of the time.

There are three types of simple sugars: glucose, fructose and lactose. Common table sugar, or sucrose, is a combination of glucose and fructose. Glucose is found in pastas, breads, cereals, etc. Fructose is found in fruits. Lactose is found in dairy products and, of course, sucrose is found in sweets. Glucose enters the blood stream immediately, triggering a large release of insulin by the pancreas. Fructose and lactose must be converted by the liver into glucose before they can enter the bloodstream. For this reason, foods containing fructose or lactose (and not glucose) tend to raise blood sugar and the body's insulin response more slowly and steadily.

The popularity of recent low-carbohydrate diets created an entire industry of low carbohydrate foods and convinced many people that all carbohydrates and sugars were bad for them. Our bodies, and our brains in particular, burn the glucose from digested carbohydrates as energy. When there aren't enough carbohydrates, they burn fat. Therefore, the low-carb diet theory goes, if you don't eat carbs, your body must burn fat as energy and you will lose weight. However, this diet ignores the fact that there are really two kinds of carbohydrates.

As with fats, there are good carbohydrates and bad carbohydrates. Renowned author Dr. William Sears has a great way of describing carbohydrates. He says, generally speaking, the carbohydrates packaged by nature (in fruits, vegetables and whole grain) are good for you and the carbohydrates packaged by a factory (in refined foods) are bad for you. When nature packages carbohydrates, it also packages fiber and protein, which slow the release of sugar into the blood stream. When a factory packages carbohydrates, it typically does not package fiber and protein and sugar is released into the bloodstream too rapidly. Another well known doctor-author, Dr. Andrew Weil, suggests that people should ignore the notion that complex carbohydrates are good and simple carbohydrates are bad. Instead, he says, people should pay attention to the glycemic index of a food because it is a much better indication of how quickly glucose is released into the bloodstream when the carbohydrate is digested. The lower the glycemic index of a food, the slower glucose is released into the bloodstream when that food is digested. According to Dr. Weil, eating a lot of high-glycemic index foods seems to be correlated with obesity, high blood pressure and adult-onset diabetes in many people.

Sugar consumption also creates sugar cravings, causing you to eat more and more sugar. When you eat a high-sugar meal, you have a sudden spike in blood-glucose level which in turn causes a hasty production and release of insulin into your blood to control the blood-glucose level. The pancreas, which produces insulin, often over-produces insulin in response because the spike in blood glucose is so severe. As a result, excess insulin remains in the bloodstream, which triggers a need for more blood-glucose to level off the insulin, and this leads to a craving for sugar. This craving is often satisfied with a high-sugar snack that starts the process all over again.

Among scientists, there exists a theory that sweets cravings also come from the body's survival instinct. In this theory, the body creates cravings for sweets because it has become programmed throughout history to "know" that sweets have a high calorie and nutrition content (fruits, for example). The body creates cravings to seek these foods out in order to have its basic calorie and nutrition needs met. Cravings in pregnant women are believed to be the body's chemical signals to serve nutritional needs. Pickles and ice cream, a cliché today, could easily be explained as the body seeking sodium from salty foods and calories and nutrition from sweet foods. Because the body is supporting a growing and changing new life, the cravings happen to surface at the same time.

Unlike the fruit that our bodies are believed to be programmed to seek out, however, modern convenience sweets are made largely of refined sugar with little or no nutritional content. Complex nutritional needs in our bodies are believed to create cravings that we now satisfy with simple, but sweet, nutrition. Those complex nutritional needs go unsatisfied, creating more cravings, and we repeat the cycle. What a goldmine these cravings are for food companies! I do not believe that there is a sinister plot to permanently deprive some undefined (and as-yet unproven) craving center in the body to keep it coming back for more, but it certainly helps to explain the enormous consumption of sugar in the U.S.

No matter how the cravings are created, people in "modern" countries like the U.K. and the U.S. have an incredible appetite for sugar. You can be sure that the "sugar lobby" in these countries spends a lot of money trying to keep the government from recommending a reduction in sugar consumption. Despite the many known health risks, the new food pyramid released by USDA in 2005 only has mild warnings against sugar consumption.

If it wasn't already clear, I recommend a diet low in refined sugar. However, I do not support the low carbohydrate diets that have become so popular. This is because, as was stated above, all carbs are *not* created equal. Fruits, vegetables and whole grains all contain carbohydrates that are health-promoting. By contrast, refined sugars contain carbohydrates that can increase blood sugar without providing the fiber and nutrients needed to prevent disease. The latter is what you need to avoid. Therefore, I recommend a low refined-sugar diet.

You can eliminate much of the refined sugar in your diet by avoiding cookies, cake, candy, chocolate, sweet pastries, ice cream, pie, sweetened soft drinks and sports drinks, sweetened cereals and fruit juices with added sugar. These processed foods are not only full of sugar, they are typically synthetically manipulated to increase shelf life so that they have very little nutrition. To produce these foods, manufacturers use chemicals and additives that are extremely unhealthy for our bodies: hydrogenated oils, preservatives, coloring agents, additives, binders, glazes, sweeteners and bleaches, to name a few. Avoid consuming these sweets and you will see your health improve in a variety of ways. Most notably, your immune system will improve and you will see the number of colds you get significantly decline.

If you are like me, however, life without the occasional sweet indulgence just isn't worth living! To be sure, I still eat sweets, but I eat them very sparingly. I typically have a small, sweet morsel one or two times per day, usually after a meal.

Only tobacco dependency has a more negative affect on human health than sugar dependency. As a result of taste-bud marketing, sugar consumption in America is at an all-time high and the range of health problems that result from it are evident in virtually every walk of life:

headaches, hormonal imbalances, hyperactivity, diabetes, hypoglycemia, heart disease, cancer, etc. Most importantly, sugar dependency suppresses the immune system, reducing the body's ability to fight against the disease processes that inevitably result from our toxic lifestyles. Having been a sugar addict myself, I can assure you that you *can* eliminate this dependency from your life. Using the system laid out for you in Part III of this book, you can overcome this degenerating addiction.

Alcohol

As most everyone knows, alcohol is a sedative and it kills brain cells, but making you sluggish and slow is not its only ill effect. Have you ever noticed the skin of people that you know who drink too much? Their skin is leathery and more wrinkled than that of other people their age. I have a couple of friends, one male and one female, who both drink a lot and have been doing it for fifteen years or so. They both look haggard and at least ten years older than everyone else their age. This is because the alcohol they drink every night is causing free radical damage throughout their bodies and their face just happens to be the area where you and I notice the damage.

Excessive drinking raises the risk of cancer of the breast, colon, liver, mouth, larynx and esophagus. It may also be linked with cancer of the pancreas and lung. Regular consumption of even a few drinks per week is associated with an increased risk of breast cancer in women. And if you smoke *and* drink, you are at a higher risk for several degenerative diseases than if you do either of these alone. For example, people who smoke *and* drink alcohol not only have a heightened risk of developing colon cancer, they tend to develop it an average of five years earlier than those who either smoked *or* drank, but did not do both.

What is that you say? Wait just wait a darn minute? You have read that alcohol is good for you? You read that red wine is good for your heart and I am a fun-stealing health-Nazi?

I have read the studies too, and it is easy to read into them what you want to see. It is true that the French have a lower rate of cancer and heart disease and it is also believed to be true that it has something to do with the red wine they drink. However, if it is indeed true, it is because of the carotenoids in the grape seeds of the grapes used to make wine, which is an element that exists in the wine along with alcohol. The alcohol in the red wine is still unhealthy for the French. And you don't have to suffer the negative effects of alcohol to get the carotenoids in your diet. Grape seed extract is available in most health food stores, pharmacies and grocery stores. (Oh yea, and grapes have grape seeds, too!)

Chemically, alcohol can be toxic to the body. The liver converts alcohol into acetaldehyde and then into acetic acid (also known as vinegar), which is harmless. However, unconverted acetaldehyde is a toxic poison to the body. Drinking alcohol to excess overburdens the liver and leaves unconverted acetaldehyde in the body, which can cause problems ranging from nausea to heart arrhythmia and palpitations.

In addition, all alcoholic drinks contain myriad compounds besides alcohol. Called congeners, these compounds come from the processes and plants used to make alcohol taste better. They include acetone, methanol, ethyl acetate, methyl ethyl ketone, histamines, prostaglandins and phytoestrogens. Methanol, for example, in larger quantities than contained in an alcoholic beverage, can cause blindness and even death in humans. Phytoestrogens are plant hormones that can generate female-like characteristics including gynocomastia (breast enlargement), in men who drink too much. Histamines are the molecules that show up in your bloodstream during an allergic response causing nasal congestion. Scientists have measured thousands of different congeners in a single alcoholic drink.

Drinking alcohol for many people is more than a habit or routine – it's a lifestyle. Many people build their social lives around alcohol and drinking in a social setting is generally expected of adults. In fact, if you don't drink alcohol in a setting where it is expected, most people assume that you are either pregnant, a recovering alcoholic, a Southern Baptist or a Mormon.

Because of the social infrastructure that supports the routine of drinking alcohol, this habit is particularly hard to alter. I know this to be true. I really enjoyed drinking and usually had a hell of a lot of fun when I drank excessively. Drinking was woven into the fabric of my social life. All of my friends drink and there is alcohol in every social setting that I attend.

The current medical position on alcohol is not to avoid it completely. The American Lung Association advises people to drink moderately, rather than give up alcohol completely, because of its protective benefits against cardiovascular disease. I take issue with this recommendation primarily because it assumes that you are going to live your life in a way that will cause cardiovascular disease.

My recommendation is different because I assume that you are going to take up a healthy lifestyle and reduce your risk of cardiovascular disease in other ways. I recommend that you drink excessively in your twenties, spend your early-thirties simultaneously reliving and regretting it, and then clean up your act.

Just kidding.

I recommend enjoying alcohol, but not doing it habitually. I recommend drinking alcohol occasionally and conservatively. If alcohol is a regular part of your daily life or if you drink more than three drinks when you do drink, your alcohol consumption is a detriment to your health. Furthermore, I suggest that people with a history of breast, colon or liver cancer in their family consider avoiding alcohol altogether except for very special occasions.

Medical Drugs
I recently saw a commercial for a new "condition" called RLS… Restless Leg Syndrome. Despite the fact that I had never heard of it, RLS appears to be so bad that it has been classified as a *syndrome*. Fortunately for the many thousands of people with agitated appendages, there is a drug called Requip from the good people at GlaxoSmithKline and Sun Pharmaceuticals. They have gotten this drug to market just in time to calm the millions of restless legs that are putting such a strain on our medical system.

For a moment, I thought the commercial was a skit on *Saturday Night Live*, poking fun at drug companies by making up an absurd condition. When the fast-talking voice at the end of the commercial listed the array of side effects from the drug, I realized that that this was a real drug from a real drug company. As discussed in an earlier section of this book, drugs are big business and consumers are made to believe that they are *good* for them.

Drug companies work hard to win the minds of doctors in order to win the wallets of their patients. On a recent visit to my doctor's office, I walked into the waiting room and felt like I had just walked onto a pharmaceutical tradeshow. There was a Levitra rock paperweight, a fancy Avandia sign-in clip board, pens logoed with Toprol XL, Namenda and Kyphon held in a Lexapro pen holder, a Nexium hand sanitizer bottle, a WelChol sign to remind you to turn off your cell phone, clocks logoed with CingulAIR and Risperdal M-Tab, a Viagra lotion dispenser and tissue box (not kidding), and a Protonix stuffed animal – and this was just in the waiting room.

The reality of medical drugs is that nearly all of them are synthetic chemicals and nearly all synthetic chemicals create adverse reactions in the human body. As has been discussed in this book, the human body is a biochemical organism which can, therefore, be modified biologically and chemically. In comparison to the complex and highly individualized chemistry of each and every human body, synthetic medical drugs are chemically simple. Targeted to a specific biochemical outcome, medical drugs lack the chemical sophistication to account for other chemical processes and reactions that inevitably result from their use. For example, a certain class of migraine headache drugs is intended to create a reaction in the body that constricts blood vessels in order to eliminate migraine headache pain. Unfortunately, the comparatively simple chemical makeup of these drugs inadvertently triggers a series of unintended biochemical processes in the complex chemistry of the human body. These "side effects" as they are called can include temperature sensitivity, muscle pain, tingling sensations, trouble swallowing, hot flashes, dizziness and even cardiac arrest. In essence, modern medicine lacks the chemical sophistication to design chemicals that *only* cause the targeted reaction.

As a result, when we take medical drugs, *other* reactions occur that are typically undesirable in the human body – many of which may be happening at a molecular or genetic level that we simply don't understand. As I have described, the accumulation of persistent synthetic chemicals and chemical processes in the human body is one of the conditions necessary for the Cumulative Effect to occur. Another condition is a weakened immune system that can't fight off the molecular and genetic defects that result from the chemical reactions going on in the human body.

Ironically, medical drugs that are potentially toxic at a molecular and genetic level are often prescribed when your immune system *is at its weakest*. Think about it: you go to the doctor when you are sick and your immune system is fighting some problem in your body. After reviewing your condition, the doctor often prescribes some type of synthetic chemical for you to take. Unfortunately, the introduction of a synthetic chemical into your body couldn't come at a worse time. The synthetic chemicals in the medical drug trigger chemical reactions that science cannot control and, naturally, one can conclude, does not fully understand. The chemicals themselves or the reactions they cause may be the source of molecular and genetic malfunctions. If they are, they are often introduced into the body when the immune system is at its weakest, unable to effectively defend itself.

Complicating things even further, every person's chemistry is different. Starting at birth, there are subtle chemical differences between people. Then, as you grow, each of us encounters a different set of chemicals in their life and environment, resulting in changes in personal chemistry. Why do you think the list of side effects for many pharmaceuticals are so long? Because adding a new chemical to a population of organisms that each has slightly different chemistry will yield different chemical reactions across that population, resulting in a long list of possible side effects. Yet drug companies treat each of us as though we are exactly the same.

Drug companies are easy targets, but medical drugs do serve a purpose. They have a role in medicine, but I think it is very different than the role they play today. However, before you read my specific recommendations, I need to be clear about your responsibilities as it relates to the information in this book and to this section in particular. I am not a physician or trained medical professional and I do not recommend that you ignore the recommendations of your doctor. Every situation is unique and before stopping medical drugs that have been prescribed to you by a medical professional, you and that medical professional need to assess the potential risks associated with stopping the drug. To be sure, you are responsible for evaluating all of your options and making an informed decision.

So, with the disclaimer out of the way, here are my recommendations regarding pharmaceuticals:

- For non-life threatening conditions, I recommend that you take medical drugs as a last resort, not a first response, to a set of symptoms. Your first response should be to take steps to help your immune system, the doctor within, fight the set of symptoms (like getting plenty of sleep, temporarily eliminating *all* refined sugar, drinking an excess of clean water and getting a variety of phytochemicals into your body from fresh fruits and vegetables). If your immune system is unable to overcome the condition by itself, then "outside help" should be considered.

- If you have a non-life-threatening condition that prevents you from living a normal life such as pain – and there exists a medical drug that can successfully eliminate the symptoms and the list of known side effects for that drug are less severe than the symptoms themselves – you should consider taking the medical drugs to address the symptoms.

- If you have a life threatening emergency and medical drugs can help you, you need to take them.

In general, I believe you should minimize medical drugs by identifying and dealing with the true *causes* of your symptoms. Medical drugs do not typically address causes. They usually only deal with symptoms. And, more often than not, the symptoms of poor health are a result of the same cause: the Cumulative Effect. If you deal with the Cumulative Effect, you can typically eliminate the symptoms that are causing you to need to take symptom-suppressing, synthetic medical drugs.

And finally, while I am again on my soap box, I recommend that you find a doctor that balances his belief in chemistry with his belief in the power of the human immune system. Don't let doctors partner with drug companies to run chemical experiments on your body. Look around you – it obviously isn't working well for anyone other than the drug companies.

Narcotics
All narcotics habits are bad for your health. Everyone knows that they are. I will not waste paper, ink and energy to tell you that.

Caffeine

I put caffeine low on the list in this chapter because recent research has not identified any long-term side effects on the human body. This has been viewed as great news for "beanies," those coffee bar groupies who always have a $6 coffee close at hand. However, caffeine is a stimulant and it is addictive. Your body develops a chemical dependency on caffeine and that is why you get a withdrawal headache when you do not have it.

Despite the studies, I recommend that you consume caffeine in moderation. Common sense says that addictive-stimulants-that-cause-withdrawal-symptoms-when-you-stop-using-them probably cause some adverse health problems. Enjoy caffeine in moderation (moderation means less than two cups – and I don't mean cauldrons, I mean cups – of caffeinated beverage per day).

	Consumption	**Quantity**
Tobacco	Never	None
Sugar	In moderation	Avoid refined sugar
Alcohol	In moderation	< 3 drinks
Medical Drugs	Only when necessary	As directed
Narcotics	Never	None
Caffeine	In moderation	Up to 2 small cups/ day

In a Nutshell: The Be In-Dependent Rules
1. Sugar, alcohol and caffeine should be consumed in moderation.
2. Minimize the use of medical drugs where appropriate by identifying and addressing the *causes* of your symptoms.
3. Avoid tobacco and narcotics altogether if you want to live a healthy life.

Chapter 8

Use Your Body

A man's health can be judged by which he takes two at a time - pills or stairs.

Joan Welsh

In addition to our ability to reason, our remarkably dexterous bodies distinguish us from other animals and have enabled us to dominate our world and virtually everything in it. Our bodies have four appendages that are attached to a torso that safely houses the vital organs inside of a protective rib cage. Our bodies have over 63 joints and can bend in many places and in many directions. They can grasp, flex, jump, hyperextend, squat, turn, kick, throw, climb, descend, pick up, put down, twist, punch, raise, lower, hang, lift, squeeze, drop and otherwise manipulate and contort in thousands of different ways. It is clear from the functionality of our bodies that they were meant to be active and used.

We are learning more and more every day that putting our bodies to use helps to prevent many of the most common degenerative diseases and health conditions. For example, regular physical activity throughout life can help protect against some cancers. Dr. Don Colbert, author of many health books including *Walking in Divine Health*, estimates that regular exercise reduces your risk of getting cancer by 65%, based on currently available statistics. For breast and prostate cancer, physical activity may help reduce cancer risk by regulating hormone levels. For colon cancer, physical activity speeds up the digestive process, shortening the exposure of the bowel lining to harmful substances that can cause the disease. And because exercise helps to maintain a healthy weight, it reduces the cancer risk associated with obesity.

Regular exercise can also dramatically reduce your risk of developing heart disease. Regular physical activity strengthens the heart muscle, reduces blood pressure, reduces LDL (bad) cholesterol levels and increases HDL (good) cholesterol, significantly reducing your risk of heart disease. Applying the other habits found in the chapters of this book will help you reduce free radicals, reduce the fat in your diet, and reduce the stress in your life, further diminishing the risk factors related to heart disease.

In addition to reducing your risk for cancer and heart disease, exercise is thought to improve brain function and, therefore, reduce the risk of some degenerative neurological disorders, particularly age-related conditions. Brain shrinkage typically starts in a person's 40's, especially in regions of the brain responsible for memory and higher cognition. Older brains process information more slowly and have difficulty switching from one task to another or multitasking.

It was long thought that mental stimulation, crossword puzzles for example, would help to keep aging brains mentally sharp, but this has been difficult to prove. According to a study released in *The Journal of Gerontology: Medical Sciences* in November, 2006, older adults who did moderate aerobic exercise for as little as three hours per week reversed their cognitive decline. In fact, the people in the study actually experienced neurogenesis – the growth of new brain cells. In only three months, the older adults studied increased their volume of grey matter (neurons) and white matter (connections between neurons). In a 2005 study published in *The Annals of Internal Medicine*, it was reported that older people who exercise three or more times per week are 30% to 40% less likely to develop Alzheimer's disease and other types of dementia. So, while the stereotype about people with big muscles being thick-headed may be true, it wasn't the exercise that made them that way! Exercise, we are learning, is good for maintaining and regenerating brain function.

Active Lifestyle, Health Fitness and Physical Fitness
Before you begin to get sweaty palms about establishing a new exercise routine in your life, let me reassure you that this chapter is *not* about becoming an aerobics instructor, a bodybuilder or a triathlete. This chapter's title is Use Your Body, and it implies something very different than simply establishing an exercise routine. Very simply, it means… *use* your body.

Healthy people are active people – at work, at home and at play. They live vigorous lives that have lead many experts to reexamine the current paradigm of exercise. The new, evolving view of exercise is to view it as the sum total of one's daily activity instead of viewing it as the hour or so spent in the gym. I think it was Raquel Welch that said, "I always take the stairs," and that is exactly the spirit to which I am referring.

I believe that there are many people who exercise regularly that would still be considered sedentary and not ever know it. They drive to work, sit all morning at their desk or in meetings, drive to lunch, sit at lunch, drive back to the office, sit at their desk all afternoon, drive home or to the gym, exercise for 45 minutes, sit for dinner, sit in front of the TV and then lie in bed and sleep until morning. Because they exercise for 45 minutes every day, they would believe that they are physically active. Although someone who exercises 45 minutes every day is more active than the majority of the population, does 23 ¼ out of 24 hours of every day sitting or laying down sound active to you? With a body that is designed to be used, does being physically motionless for 97% of your life sound active? It isn't.

The human body was not designed to be left idling. When it is left unused 97% of the time, the human body atrophies, becomes brittle and fragile and ages prematurely. "Use Your Body" means more than exercising three times per week for thirty minutes (although that is a tremendous start). It means getting up and being active, often. It means engaging in physical activities on the weekend like gardening and home improvement. It means being active in the evening at home. And it means being active at work, no matter what your vocation.

Regular vigorous exercise such as running, cycling or lifting weights has numerous proven benefits, however maintaining such a program can be tough for many people, especially those who are sedentary. Fortunately, numerous studies now show that a dramatic improvement in health can be made from just a small increase in activity, particularly for those people who are inactive. There is an emerging notion of *health fitness* that is somewhat different than the notion of *physical fitness* to which we have become accustomed. Consider the following:

- In 2006, the journal *Diabetes Care* showed that those who did moderate exercise added nearly 2.5 years to life expectancy versus those who were sedentary.
- A 1999 study of more than 800 residents of Kings County, Washington, showed dramatic health benefits among those who gardened or walked for a total of just one hour per week, translating to about a 70% lower risk of dying from sudden cardiac arrest.
- A 2004 report by researchers in Sweden showed that adults who only exercised once per week were 40% less likely to die during the study period than those who were sedentary.

- According to Harvey B. Simon, M.D., the author of *The No Sweat Exercise Plan*, exercising for 30 minutes just six days per month can lower the mortality rate by 43%.
- Dr. Mike Rozien and Dr. Mehmet Oz, authors of *YOU: The Owner's Manual*, believe that sixty minutes of cardiovascular exercise per week (what they call stamina exercise - three twenty minute sessions done at 80% of your maximum heart rate), is all you need to achieve the longevity benefits of exercise.

A program designed around the traditional notion of *physical fitness* might include running sprints at a track, lifting weights and swimming laps in a 50 meter pool. A *health fitness* program, by contrast, could include taking the stairs to your office, cleaning the house and walking the dog every day. Recent studies have shown that the health benefits of exercise kick in with the first 1,000 calories burned each week. In other words, there is growing evidence that one can achieve health fitness by exercising through only 140 calories per day, and that is attainable by any person. Baring a physical condition that leaves you motionless, health fitness can be achieved without having to commit to a rigorous exercise program.

Check out the amount of calories burned in a half hour for some common exercises and daily activities, based on a 150-pound person.

Activity	Calories Burned Per ½ hour - Man	Calories Burned Per ½ hour – Woman
Golf, baseball, cleaning house, bicycling (< 10 mph) , walking (3.5 mph)	140 – 150	110 – 120
Walking (4.5 mph), weight lifting (vigorous effort), swimming (slow freestyle laps), aerobics, gardening	220 – 250	175 – 200
Jogging (6 mph), jumping rope, bicycling (> 10 mph)	290 – 375	230 – 300
Running, racquetball, cross country skiing	450	370

While living an active lifestyle or achieving health fitness can cause tremendous improvements in the health of previously inactive people, I need to be careful not to cause you to conclude that they provide the same benefits as the traditional *physical fitness* programs. As stated above, *the health benefits of exercise kick in with the first 1,000 calories burned each week.* However, physical fitness tends to create greater health benefits than an active lifestyle or health fitness in areas such as cardiovascular condition, bone density and weight management. Because we find ourselves particularly prone to degenerative conditions such as atherosclerosis, osteoporosis, obesity and cancer, I believe that the incremental benefits provided by physical fitness are important to understand and strive for.

Physical fitness is defined differently by different groups and its definition has varied over time. It is defined on Wikipedia as "the body's ability to function efficiently and effectively in work and leisure activities, to be healthy, to resist hypokinetic diseases (conditions that occur from a sedentary lifestyle), and to meet emergency situations. Fitness can also be divided into five categories: aerobic fitness, muscular strength, muscular endurance, flexibility, and body composition."

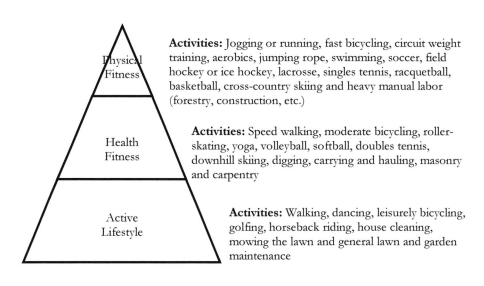

Physical Fitness

Activities: Jogging or running, fast bicycling, circuit weight training, aerobics, jumping rope, swimming, soccer, field hockey or ice hockey, lacrosse, singles tennis, racquetball, basketball, cross-country skiing and heavy manual labor (forestry, construction, etc.)

Health Fitness

Activities: Speed walking, moderate bicycling, roller-skating, yoga, volleyball, softball, doubles tennis, downhill skiing, digging, carrying and hauling, masonry and carpentry

Active Lifestyle

Activities: Walking, dancing, leisurely bicycling, golfing, horseback riding, house cleaning, mowing the lawn and general lawn and garden maintenance

Since nearly all of us in the "modern" world are theoretically sedentary, adopting an active lifestyle will result in important gains in overall health. However, because only physical fitness can cause meaningful health improvements in areas that we are particularly prone to degenerative diseases, an active lifestyle and health fitness should be viewed as the foundation on which physical fitness can be achieved. Therefore, I recommend that sedentary people set a goal of becoming active; active people set a goal of achieving health fitness (burning at least 140 calories every day through an active lifestyle); and active, healthy people set a goal of achieving and maintaining physical fitness (as defined earlier). Refer to the graphic on the previous page for examples of the types of activities that you might explore in the various categories of exercise.

Types of Exercise
Physical activity of any kind requires the exertion of energy that being idle does not. Being sedentary is the path of least resistance and the longer that path has been followed, the deeper the rut is to climb out of. Therefore, it is essential to create a fitness program that is appealing to you. If you choose activities that are appealing to you, you will be motivated to break the routine of inactivity and consistently overcome the mental barriers created by the anticipation of exercise.

Whether your current goal is an active lifestyle, health fitness or physical fitness, I recommend that you include some cardiovascular activity, resistance activity and stretching in your routine. By combining these three types of activity and varying the exercises within each activity, you can condition your whole body. In addition, the variety of activities that you will undertake in the program that I recommend will keep things interesting, helping to prevent you from falling back into physical inactivity.

Cardiovascular Exercise - The terms cardiovascular exercise, aerobic exercise and cardiorespiratory fitness are all synonymous. This kind of exercise requires large muscle movement over a sustained period of time and elevating your heart rate to some percent of its maximum level. Examples include walking, running, cycling, swimming, aerobics, dance, rowing, cross country skiing and any other repetitious activity that can be performed over an extended period of time.

Cardiovascular exercise has numerous benefits including increased heart and lung function and efficiency, decreased blood pressure, decreased body fat, increased HDL (good) cholesterol, decreased LDL (bad) cholesterol, and increased capillary density and blood flow to active muscles. On top of this, cardiovascular exercise has also shown to decrease tension, anxiety and depression. All of these benefits combine to help lower your risk of cardiovascular disease by reducing risk factors like obesity, hypertension, and high blood cholesterol.

Many people believe that the heart muscle wears out and use this as an excuse <u>not</u> to do cardiovascular exercise. I've actually had friends tell me, "I don't know why you people run/cycle/exercise all the time. All you are doing is wearing out your heart." This is an often used as an excuse for not exercising. In reality, the opposite is true. Cardiovascular exercise will actually increase the life of your heart.

While cardiovascular exercise does dramatically increase your heart rate during exercise, the strengthening of the heart muscle that results from regular exercise increases the efficiency of the heart muscle, allowing it to push more blood with each pump (beat). By pushing more blood with each pump, the body needs fewer pumps (beats) per minute to meet its oxygen/ nutrition needs.

Let's do the math: If your resting heart rate was 70 beats per minute (bpm) and you were to do aerobic exercise three times per week – raising your resting heart rate from 70 bpm to 125 bpm for a half hour each time – you would add 1,650 additional heart beats per day and ~260,000 additional heart beats per year.

If, however, as a result of this exercise regimen, you reduced your resting heart rate from 70 beats per minute to 65 beats per minute (which is very realistic), you would have reduced your heart rate by 7,200 beats per day and ~2.6 million beats per year. If you subtract the increase in heart rate caused by the exercise regimen, you are still reducing your total heart beats by over 2.3 million per year. And, if you kept up this program for thirty years, you would reduce the number of beats that your heart would be required to pump by over 70 million heart beats (nearly two full years of heart beats at 70 bpm)! So, if it is true, that your heart muscle wears out and your heart only has so many beats in its useful life, you actually *need* to do regular cardiovascular exercise to extend your heart's life!

Because of the myriad of benefits that result from regular cardiovascular exercise, I recommend that you elevate your heart rate into its target heart rate range for at least 20 minutes three or more times per week. To find your target heart rate range for exercise, subtract your age from 220.

Then, multiply that number by .65 and .8 to get the low and high numbers of your target heart rate range for exercise. For example, the target heart rate for a 48-year old would be 112 to 138 (220 - 48 = 172, 172 x .65 = 112, 172 x .8 = 138). So, when a 48-year old person does cardiovascular exercise, he should try to achieve a heart rate of between 112 and 138 and sustain it for at least 20 minutes to achieve the maximum cardiovascular benefit.

Resistance Exercise - The terms resistance exercise, strength training and weight lifting are all synonymous. Resistance exercise increases muscle strength by repeatedly pitting the muscles against a weight or force. The muscle cells adapt to the extra workload by getting bigger and using more nerve cells to help the muscles contract. Resistance training can include free weights such as barbells and dumbbells, weight machines, resistance bands and even your own body weight.

Resistance exercise has a number of benefits outside of muscle size and strength that are very important to overall health. They include increased bone density and strength, reduced body fat, a lowered heart rate and blood pressure, and a reduced risk of developing some conditions like diabetes. Resistance training even increases your metabolism, allowing you to burn more calories when at rest. Research has shown that regular resistance training can increase your Basal Metabolic Rate (basically the rate at which your body "runs" when idling) by up to 15%.

Because obesity, osteoporosis, heart disease and diabetes have become common, chronic conditions in our society, and because resistance exercise provides health benefits that other forms of exercise do not, it should be viewed as an essential component of any exercise program. I recommend that you mix resistance exercise into your exercise regimen at least two times per week for a minimum of 30 minutes per session.

Be cautious not to overdo it if you are a beginner or if you have not done resistance exercise for more than four weeks. Your muscles can become sore from the build up of lactic acid and you may even injure yourself. Also, make sure that you warm up your muscles by stretching and doing some brief cardiovascular exercise before you begin a resistance exercise session.

Choose 8-10 basic exercises that cover the major muscle groups of your body and choose a weight that you can lift between eight and 12 times with some effort for each exercise. Make sure to study the correct body positioning (form) for each exercise to reduce the risk of injury. Note that you do not have to do every exercise during every session. Some people split their routines into upper body exercises one day and lower body exercises another. Still others do push exercises (presses, squats, etc.) one day and pull exercises another (pull ups, curls, etc.). What is most important is that you receive the health benefits of resistance training, which come from regular resistance exercises for each muscle group in your body.

There are a number of excellent books and websites devoted to strength training exercises. I personally recommend www.crossfit.com, but it should be noted that Crossfit is for those seeking to reach the level of physical fitness on the pyramid above.

Stretching - Stretching is a vital part of any exercise program and should be viewed as being just as important as cardiovascular and resistance exercise. As you age, your muscles tighten and range of motion in the joints can be minimized. This can put a damper on a vigorous lifestyle and make you more prone to injuries.

Stretching reduces muscle tension and fatigue, improves circulation and joint health, increases range of motion and, most importantly, decreases the likelihood of injuries from physical activity. Regular stretching increases the length of both your muscles and tendons, which means your limbs and joints can move further before an injury occurs. In addition, an effective warm up that includes stretching will help to raise body temperature, increase blood flow and promote oxygen supply to the muscles. It will also help to prepare the mind, muscles, tendons and joints for the physical activity to come.

Everyone can learn to stretch, regardless of age or flexibility. It is a very natural activity for the body. You might notice when you wake up or when you have been sitting in a particular position for a long time, you stretch unconsciously. Stretching is the simplest of the three types of physical activities.

I recommend that you follow a 10 – 15 minute stretching and warm up routine before any cardiovascular or resistance exercise. Begin with common stretches of major muscle groups and pay particular attention to stretching and warming up your back and your hamstrings as they are both particularly prone to injury. If you are unfamiliar with common stretches, there are dozens of books on the subject and the Internet can serve as a very effective reference as well.

Using Your Body

A consistent regimen of cardiovascular exercise, resistance training and stretching provides numerous benefits: It lowers your heart rate and blood pressure, potentially prolonging your heart's life. It pumps oxygen-rich blood to the cells and tissues of your body providing nourishment. It keeps weight under control, reduces body fat and increases lean muscle mass. It detoxifies the body through perspiration. It keeps your digestion and waste elimination on schedule if done routinely. It improves blood cholesterol levels. It increases your body's metabolic rate. It increases the range of motion of your muscles and joints. It improves sleep, releases tension and reduces stress. It increases bone strength and density and prevents bone loss. It boosts energy and causes the release of endorphins in the brain promoting a sense of well-being. It establishes a good example for children, family and friends to follow. And, in older people, it helps maintain quality of life and independence longer.

For all its benefits, however, making exercise a routine is something that most people have repeatedly tried and repeatedly failed to do. In fact, I have only seen one other successful method (other than this one) for getting people to make exercise a permanent part of their life: a doctor who looks them in the eye and tells them that they are killing themselves. There are a million psychological justifications for not exercising regularly, but they all stem from the same obstacle: exercise creates discomfort and our bodies naturally prefer comfort to discomfort.

Using the methods for building habits described in Part III of this book, I believe that you can start or stop any habit, even this one. Because exercise is particularly difficult to maintain over time (and because I can't throw on a stethoscope and look each one of you in the eyes and tell you that you are killing yourself in order to motivate you), here are some tips I have found very helpful over the 24 years that I have maintained a regular exercise program:

If you are just starting, take it slowly. This is for two important reasons. First, you could hurt yourself by trying to do too much too soon. If this is new for you, your heart, lungs and muscles are not accustomed to the workload that regular exercise will put on them and you run a risk of injury. However, this is the less important reason because, while painful, injury is typically temporary and you can return to your routine when you heal.

The second, and far more important, reason that you don't want to overdo a new activity or exercise regimen is that you run a very high risk of burn-out. When I was younger, I used to work out at health clubs. Every January, the club would be packed with droves of New Year's resolution-ers wearing shiny new sweat suits and spotless running shoes. They would turn up in packs with that "I'm-committed-to-looking-like-the-guy-on-the-cover-of-Men's-Fitness-magazine" look in their eyes. They would work every machine in the place and then hop on the treadmill, the bike and finally the elliptical trainer. As they stammered out of the health club, dripping in sweat, one after another, we knew that the gym would again be ours by January 20th. They set the exercise routine bar so high that the physical stress of exercise outweighed the emotional stress of being out of shape. Eventually, they quit and fell right back into the rut that they had been in for years – that of doing nothing.

Don't let that happen to you. This is an important habit. Take it slowly. By slowly increasing the duration, frequency and intensity of your activity or exercise, you will ensure that you don't injure yourself or burn out.

Exercise/ be active at the same time. This might be the single biggest factor in making exercise a permanent part of your life. Doing something at the same time nearly every day, over and over again, causes your body to expect, and often crave, that stimulus at that time. This helps a lot when you might otherwise lack the motivation for exercise.

Figure out what time regularly works for your schedule and make sure it is a time when you consistently feel energetic. This consistent repetition will help you to create a habit of activity. If you sense that this time is beginning to be a problem for some reason, find a new time.

Figure out what you need to keep you interested. I watch my favorite TV programs and browse my favorite magazines in between sets while I lift weights. I also bring along my favorite cereal or fruit to snack on between sets. When I run or cycle, I listen to my favorite music and I wear good-looking exercise clothes because nice clothes make us all feel good.

Don't make being active harder than it has to be by making your exercise uninteresting. Make it as enjoyable as possible by surrounding yourself with things that you like. Bring your favorite magazine, wear clothes that make you look good, load up a digital music player with your favorite music, bring something along to snack on, etc.

Find the right place to exercise/ be active. Surroundings are important. I have worked out in gyms and run and ridden my bike all over the place. I enjoyed the diversity. However, when I had kids, it became more important for me to spend as much time as I could with them. It's convenient, comfortable and safe to work out at home and it allows your family to see you being active, which sets a good example for them. .

However, working out or being active at home is not for everyone. Some people find it much more motivating to go to a health club, a high school track, or to a local park. The bottom line is this: don't be afraid to experiment with different settings in order to determine the surroundings that suit you best.

Ensure variety. Variety helps to keep an active lifestyle from becoming dull and boring. For example, I follow an exercise program called the three/one split. That is, I exercise for three consecutive days, alternating resistance and cardiovascular exercise (both with stretching), and then take a day off. In addition to alternating between the two, I utilize a variety of resistance and cardiovascular exercises.

After experimenting with various routines for the last 25 years, I have found this type of program to be the most sustainable, which is really the point. By alternating cardiovascular and resistance exercise, my routine stays fresh and interesting. Think about what will keep your attention off of your exertion – competitive sports, team sports, exercising outside, water sports, socializing, exercise as transportation – and then consider what you can fit into your lifestyle, schedule and budget. As long as you exercise enough to meet your goal (a calorie goal, for example), the amount of time you log being active every day isn't that important. What is important is that you are consistently exercising your cardiovascular system and your musculo-skeletal system. If you want to lose weight more rapidly or increase muscle tone, size or strength, simply increase the duration and/or intensity of your workouts.

Get out! In developed countries, we spend far more time inside than our ancestors did and we have lost our connection with the earth. You should try to get at least half of your exercise outside.

Today, it is common for dermatologists to tell you to stay out of the sun and that encourages many people to stay inside. However, sunlight is critical to human health. Our skin produces vitamin D, a vitamin important for immune function, from contact with sunlight. Many groups of people in primitive cultures around the world spend considerably more time in direct sunlight than those people living in developed countries (who work indoors all of the time). So why is the rate of skin cancer astronomically higher in people living in developed countries than in people living in primitive cultures? It certainly isn't the exposure to sunlight. Some theorize that it is other factors such as a poor diet that make a person susceptible to skin cancer from the harmful UV rays of the sun. People living in primitive cultures have diets rich in phytonutrient-containing fruits and vegetables. It is believed that these phytonutrients block the harmful effects of UV rays.

So, don't be afraid of the sun if you have a healthy diet. Eat well and get outside to enjoy the earth! You should use exercise as an excuse to spend more time outside.

Set a goal. Do you want to become stronger? Do you want to lose 20 pounds? Do you want to increase muscle tone in your stomach? Do you want to complete a 5k, 10k, half-marathon or marathon? Do you just want to get into your old pants or look good in a swimsuit?

Simply being healthy isn't motivation enough for some people. To really get motivated, you may need to set a goal. Goal setting and planning can be a complicated process if you allow it to be. The most important element is setting an achievable goal for yourself and writing it down somewhere you will see it every day. You will be surprised at how it motivates you in conjunction with the other elements described here.

If you aren't in the mood (and you have been fairly consistent lately), don't do it. Exercising when you are not in the mood is not enjoyable. It is a chore. As humans, we unconsciously avoid that which is not enjoyable and this will ultimately undermine our motivation to exercise.

When I lollygag around while getting my exercise clothes on, distracted by something else, debating about what exercises I do and don't want to do, going through excuses in my mind about skipping this day, I recognize that I am not in the right frame of mind and I skip that day. I don't beat myself up over it. I just skip it and know that it was the best thing for me. Many times our bodies are telling us that they are too tired to go through what we are planning to put them through. So, listen to your body and skip.

If you get in a rut, change. It happens to everyone. If you find that you are bored with your exercise routine and you begin to dread it, change the exercises and try something physical that you've never tried before. Change the gym you attend or the route you rollerblade. Change the goal from weight loss to muscle tone or from distance to speed. Change the surroundings by trying out that new MP3 player while you use the elliptical trainer or if you workout alone, try exercising with a partner.

Take steps to avoid injury. Most exercise-related injuries will force you to take some time off from exercise. For many people, that short time off is enough to cause them to slip back into their sedentary ways.

Unfortunately, minor injuries can be somewhat common when you don't stretch, warm up and use good technique. As discussed previously, cold muscles injure easily when they are made to do something that they are not designed to do or forced into vigorous use without warming them up. To avoid injury, always stretch and warm up for 10 – 15 minutes before you exercise and always use proper technique. For cardiovascular exercises like jogging or cycling, this means starting with 5 – 10 minutes of exercise at a slower than training pace followed by 5 – 10 minutes of stretching. For resistance exercises like weight training, this means starting your routine with 10 – 15 minutes of light lifting and stretching and following proper form during every set and repetition. It only takes an instant to become injured when you are too hurried to warm up or contorting your body to do something it shouldn't.

I have found these tips to be helpful in maintaining an exercise routine over time. However you do it, just do it. No matter when you start, exercise improves your health.

Important Note: Some people should consult a medical professional before they begin an exercise program. See your doctor or other healthcare provider if you are a male older than 45 or a female over 55 and have not been regularly active. Regardless of your age, if you have two or more of the following risk factors, consult a medical professional before starting an exercise program:

- High blood pressure
- Heart condition or a history of stroke
- Family history of early onset heart disease
- High cholesterol
- Diabetes
- You currently smoke
- You've developed chest pain or discomfort within the last month
- You feel extremely breathless or dizzy after mild exertion
- Your doctor said that you have bone, joint or muscle problems that could be made worse by the proposed physical activity

If none of these is true for you, you can begin a gradual, sensible program of increased activity tailored to your needs. If you feel any of the physical symptoms listed above when you start your exercise program, contact a medical professional right away. If one or more of the above is true for you, an exercise-stress test may be used to help plan an exercise program that is right for you.

In a Nutshell: The Use Your Body Rules
1. Increase your activity level. It is believed that the health benefits of exercise occur during the first 1,000 calories burned per week. Get up and move!
2. Be consistent. Getting regular exercise is more important than the actual duration of the exercise sessions themselves.
3. Do all three. Every exercise program at every level of fitness should include a combination of cardiovascular exercise, resistance exercise and stretching.

4. Emphasize variety. Vary your exercises to ensure that you are exercising your whole body, to keep things interesting, and to prevent overuse injuries.

A Word about the 8 Habits of Healthy People

If you are beginning to worry about the challenge of adopting these habits, don't. There is an activity in Part III of this book that will help you prioritize the habits that you need to adopt and a simple approach to help you adopt them and make them a routine part of your life. In addition, there is an entire website (www.habitsofhealth.com) devoted to helping you adopt The 8 Habits of Healthy People with an abundance of great resources.

Chapter 9

Carry the Right Weight

Gluttony is the source of all our infirmities, and the fountain of all our diseases. As a lamp is choked by a superabundance of oil, a fire extinguished by excess of fuel, so is the natural health of the body destroyed by intemperate diet.

Robert Burton

I once went to a University of Michigan football game. The Michigan Wolverines play in a stadium the fans call "The Big House" because it holds over 100,000 fans (107,501 to be exact). Well, actually, they call it The Big House because it holds about 5,000 more fans than the nearest rival college football stadium, Neyland Stadium at the University of Tennessee. For a college football fan like me, seeing a game in The Big House is a real treat.

As I arrived at my seat before kickoff, everyone was standing. I worked my way down the aisle to my seat number and squeezed in next to a couple of rather husky Midwestern ladies in navy blue and maize. Immediately, and I mean immediately after kickoff, the entire stadium of 107,500 people dropped to their metal bench stadium seats like a rock. I marveled at the remarkably efficient organization of these fans and bent my knees and began to lower myself down to be seated.

My descent into my seat was abruptly halted by something that I was not expecting – two rather large thighs, one covered in taut denim and the other in tightly-stretched navy blue cotton. I shot up, surprised, and spun around to look at my seat. There, between the two thighs of my husky seat neighbors, was just enough room for the number "11" painted on the metal bleacher. In that moment, I realized what every Michigan fan knew that I did not: that the synchronized sitting was not a feat of organization, but a race to get in contact with the bench to lay claim to enough metal for both cheeks. The University of Michigan didn't build a bigger stadium to fit all those fans – they simply squeeze more in per square foot than the other guys.

Suffice it to say, I was a quick study. After big plays, I made it down to my seat faster than my neighbors on most occasions. But, as I soon discovered, this was not always the winning move, believe me. As I played this game of up and down that most Michigan fans didn't mind and seemed to do involuntarily, it occurred to me that the University of Michigan based their seat spacing on the width of a normal-weight person. Given the population in this stadium and, frankly, throughout most of the United States, this was either a poor design or an intentional oversight.

According to the National Institutes of Health, nearly 62% of people living in the United States are overweight and nearly 30% are obese. Assuming that these numbers hold true in Michigan, and I am confident that they do, it means that nearly 67,000 people in the stadium that day were overweight and nearly 33,000 of them were obese. With these statistics in mind, I have concluded that it is technically accurate to say that The Big House "holds" 107,501, but it certainly doesn't "seat" 107,501. If the average overweight person is 15% larger than the normal-weight person, the stadium probably only "seats" about 97,000!

Who is Overweight and who is Obese?
Despite how generic they sound, the terms "overweight" and "obese" are actually medical terms defined by a standard measure called the body mass index (BMI), a ratio of weight to height. The medical community says that people with a BMI between 25 and 29, are overweight and people with a BMI of 30 or greater are obese. Three out of every five Americans have a BMI 25 or higher and three out of ten have a BMI of 30 or greater.

To calculate your BMI, divide your weight in pounds by your height in inches twice, and multiply by 703 (Weight in pounds ÷ Height in inches ÷ Height in inches x 703 = BMI). If you live in a country that uses the metric system, divide your weight in kilograms by your height in meters twice to get your body mass index (Weight in kilograms ÷ Height in meters ÷ Height in meters = BMI). You are deemed to be "normal" if your BMI is between 18.5 and 24.9. If your BMI is below 18.5, you are deemed "underweight." If your BMI is between 25 and 29.9, you are "overweight" and if it is over 30 you are deemed to be "obese." I think that BMI is directionally accurate, but it can be deceiving on the margins, especially for athletes with a higher than average amount of muscle mass.

Another common measure is the waist-to-hip ratio (WHR). To determine if you have a healthy WHR, use a measuring tape to measure the circumference of your hips at the widest part of your buttocks. Then measure your waist at the smaller circumference of your natural waist, usually just above the belly button.

To determine the ratio, divide your waist measurement by your hip measurement. Research shows that people with "apple-shaped" bodies (with more weight around the waist) face more health risks than those with "pear-shaped" bodies who carry more weight around the hips. A WHR of 0.7 for women and 0.9 for men have been shown to correlate strongly with general health. If you are a woman and your ratio is greater than .8 or you are a man and your ratio is greater than .95, you may be at risk for health problems such as coronary artery disease.

The United States of Fat People

Obesity has become a significant health problem in the developed world. Former U.S. President Bill Clinton feels that it is the single biggest problem facing the United States and has made curtailing the obesity epidemic in America the emphasis of his post-presidential public life. The statistics on the weight problem in the United States support Clinton's concern.

- The number of obese people grew 300% between 1980 and 2006.
- Three out of 10 children are overweight and 8 out of 10 adults over 25 are overweight.
- Over 40 million workdays are lost annually because of obesity-related health problems.
- Over 60 million physician office visits per year are a result of obesity-related health problems and medical expenses attributable to obesity reached $75 billion in 2003.
- There has been a 76% increase in Type II diabetes in adults 30-40 yrs old since 1990 and 80% of type II diabetes is related to obesity.
- Cardiovascular disease is the nation's leading killer and 70% of cardiovascular disease is related to obesity.

America is not alone in her gluttony. Other developed western countries are seeing their populations grow ever-fatter too. According to the health select committee of the House of Commons in Great Brittan, "Obesity will soon supersede tobacco as the greatest cause of premature death in

[Great Britain]. It is staggering to realize that on present trends, half of all children in England in 2020 could be obese."

Make no mistake though, obesity is not an accident. It is not sudden. It is actually quite sneaky and quiet.

Weight gain is the result of eating more calories than you burn. The human body stores excess calories as fat in order to prevent starvation – a common challenge 100 years ago, but no longer physiologically necessary. We don't have seasonal shortages of food like our ancient ancestors did. Today, we tend to have too much food and we overeat all year round. Without adequate activity and exercise, modern people accumulate those excess calories day after day. As a result, weight, in the form of fat, is hung on our bodies pound after pound, year after year, until you look down one day and you can't see your...

I have a doctor friend who is a urologist. He says that grown men come into his office on a fairly regular basis complaining of a condition transcribed onto their chart as "shrinking penis." After reading "shrinking penis" on a chart while preparing to see a patient, he knows before opening the door that he will see an obese man sitting there. He has them pull down their pants and stand in front of a mirror. He then has them pull back the fat pad that has accumulated at the base of their penis revealing, in all its glory, the penis they knew from their younger days.

My doctor friend then asks his patients, "Is this what your penis used to look like?"

"Yes! Yes, that's what it looked like," they say in amazement.

"Lose 50 to 70 pounds and your penis will grow back," he chides them.

How Did We Get So Fat?
Good question. How did we get so fat? For starters, the diet in the developed world has changed dramatically over the last several decades. In developed countries, there is now an abundance of convenient, packaged foods of all shapes, sizes and tastes. These manufactured foods, foods that have been processed in a factory, do not fulfill the nutritional needs of the human body as well as nature's foods do. So, we have to eat

more calories of manufactured food, on average, to satisfy the cravings that our nutritional needs create.

The manufactured-food diet typically consists of nutrient-poor processed foods such as white bread, pasta, potato chips, crackers and cereals, high fat foods like pork, ground beef and cheese, and sugar-laden foods like jams, cookies, cereals, cake, brownies and ice cream. And, when fruit, vegetables and grains are eaten, they have typically had the nutrients cooked or processed out. So, on this diet, even though you've eaten, you're still craving (nutrient-starved). You turn to nutrient-poor, taste-rich, convenience foods and the cycle repeats itself over and over and over.

However, that is only part of the story. There were a series of lifestyle changes that took place around 1980 that made us more sedentary and when overeating combined with inactivity, waistlines balloon. Throughout the 1960's and 1970's, obesity rates in the United States hovered around 15%. With the 1980's, Americans experienced an increase in suburban sprawl combined with the introduction of cable television and the eventual introduction of computers. People became increasingly sedentary and dependent on transportation. By 2002, obesity in the U.S. had reached 30%.

The combination of a diet based largely on manufactured food and a more sedentary lifestyle is what has caused the incredible increase in obesity in the developed world. I suppose that the profit motive of food companies played a role, too (larger portions, for example), but nothing has had a more dramatic impact than these two factors. Diet and lifestyle have changed dramatically over the last 30 years and all you have to do is go to a public place to see it. Everyone is fat. In fact, fit people look out of place.

Weight Problem = Health Problems
Weight problems cause very real and very severe health problems. Many of the most prevalent chronic health problems in the developed world are prevalent because of the obesity epidemic. And those health conditions commonly associated with being overweight are growing at an astronomical rate.

One startling example is Type II diabetes. Some 16 million people have Type II diabetes today and the number is expected to double by 2025. Obesity is a major risk factor and the likely cause of the dramatic rise expected. Interestingly, Type II diabetes was previously known as Adult Onset Diabetes, but it had to be renamed because so many young people began developing the disease. This happened because the risk factors that cause the disease, like obesity and physical inactivity, are now commonly found among younger people.

In addition to Type II diabetes, being overweight is a risk factor for high blood pressure, heart disease, stroke, kidney failure, high blood cholesterol or other lipid disorders and many types of cancer (breast, colon, endometrium, gallbladder, esophagus, pancreas and kidney). Being overweight can also cause sleep apnea, gallstones, chronic back pain and osteoarthritis in weight bearing joints. In addition, although overweight and obese people can be happy with their weight, in many people it creates self-esteem problems and depression that feed the cycle of overeating and remaining sedentary.

Big Kids

Today, twice as many children are overweight as in 1980. Why? Simply because they are sedentary and eating poorly. Think about it. There are 300 more channels of television now and thousands more combinations of conveniently packaged sugar and fat than 30 years ago.

Being overweight as a child not only creates a myriad of health risks later in life like cardiovascular disease, diabetes and cancer, but it also affects the self-esteem and confidence of young people. Society labels fat people as unattractive and believing that you are unwanted and ugly as a child creates tragic and lifelong battles with insecurity and its many behavior manifestations.

If you have young children, you can help them maintain a healthy weight by utilizing many of the ideas in this book. However, it starts with you. Children of overweight parents are twice as likely to be overweight themselves and this isn't a genetic problem – it's an environmental one. Overweight families all tend to be sedentary and all tend to eat poorly. Because your children are going to look to you as their role model, you have to set the example of healthy habits. They need to see you exercising and eating the right foods and portions before they will embrace it for themselves.

Carrying the Right Weight

Ads for expensive exercise equipment and special diets can make healthy living seem complicated and difficult to maintain. However, the truth is that there is no great secret to achieving the weight you want. It really is as simple as balancing the calories you consume with the calories that you burn. When that doesn't happen, you gain weight.

To shed weight, most people turn to the latest diet craze. Weight loss diets are thought to have first become popular in the 19th century. In the 1830's, a Presbyterian minister named Sylvester Graham, who later gave his name to the Graham cracker, recommended a bland diet to cure gluttony and immorality among his parishioners. His followers grew in number until they were described as frail and rumors of mass starvation surfaced. Over the next 175 years, dieters tried a variety of diets including Helen Rubenstein's Grapefruit Diet, the Weight Watchers calorie-counting diet, the Slim Fast liquid diet, the high protein Scarsdale Diet, the tropical fruit Beverly Hills Diet, the Cambridge low-calorie liquid diet, and the low-carb/low-fat South Beach Diet. And, in 1997, cardiologist Dr. Robert Atkins' diet book (originally published in the 1970's) was reissued popularizing a low carbohydrate approach to dieting.

Which diet do I recommend? Atkins, South Beach, The Zone, Sugar Busters, Weight Watchers, Jenny Craig, Scotch & Beef Jerky? None of the above. Overall, my advice on weight management is very simple: don't go on a diet. A diet, by definition, is temporary. It involves sudden, drastic changes in eating or lifestyle. People endure a routine that is not natural or habitual to them because they are motivated to look good and feel better about themselves. Dieters never internalize and adopt the diet routine because they know it is temporary (not that they could because it is often so unnatural). As a result, when people come off of a diet, they go right back into their habitual routines that made them overweight in the first place. Then, when they are overweight again, along comes a new diet plan and the cycle repeats itself. Unless you are the consumer products company selling the diet food or the author of the diet book, this cycle is futile.

More importantly, weight loss diets are intended to help people lose weight. They are not intended to help people become healthier. Many of the tenets of popular diets, both old and new, actually work to undermine your overall health. In most diets, there are drastic changes in the content and nutrients of the diet causing sudden shifts in the body's chemistry.

So, though weight loss diets may make you look good, the results tend to be temporary and often undermine your overall health.

According to Robert Pritikin of the Pritikin Longevity Center, scientists have studied what makes us feel full and satisfied enough to stop eating. Their conclusion, he says, is simple. We stop eating when our stomachs are full [and our nutrient cravings are nourished]. Therefore, the solution to weight management is simple, Pritikin says. Don't try to starve yourself. Go ahead and fill your stomach so you feel satisfied, but fill it with foods that are bulky but have a low calorie density (just like our prehistoric ancestors). Calorie-dense foods such as nuts, meat, breads and dairy products contain more calories per cubic inch in our stomachs than do low density foods such as fruits and vegetables. If you have to fill your stomach up to feel satisfied, you should fill it with low density foods if you are trying to lose weight.

To control your weight, you should also eat more often according to Pritikin. He suggests three smaller meals and two snacks (breakfast, mid-morning snack, lunch, mid-afternoon snack, dinner). Going hungry causes your brain to believe you are in starvation and triggers a slow down in your body's metabolism to reserve calories. A slower metabolism that burns fewer calories in a day inhibits your weight loss. In addition, starvation stimulates your body's prehistoric instinct to seek out calorie-dense foods, creating cravings that an apple or broccoli simply won't satisfy like high-calorie foods such as bread, peanut butter, meat and cheese will. And, when you do finally give in and stuff yourself, your body will store most of those calories as fat because it still believes it is in starvation. Frequent eating of the right foods keeps the body's metabolism high, burning more calories, and helping to prevent the urges, temptations and cravings that are hard for all of us to resist.

Also, don't skip meals, especially breakfast. Eating in the morning will give you the energy you need and will minimize hunger during the day, which will help you avoid overeating. Try not to go for more than four or five hours without eating (except when you are asleep at night). Being famished at mealtimes may hinder your ability to make healthy choices, as well as trigger overeating. If you do splurge with an unhealthy or rich meal, try to balance it out with healthy or light eating the rest of the day.

Lastly, do not unnaturally avoid or overdo any of the macronutrients – protein, fat and carbohydrates. A lot has been said about carbohydrate consumption and fat consumption as it relates to dieting. The low-carb diet, for example, was a phenomenal commercial success in large part due to dieter's ability to lose weight without feeling hungry. By 2004, $2.6 billion in low carbohydrate diet products had been sold. However, because the low-carb diet emphasized protein, it tended to sharply increase LDL (bad) cholesterol and its attractiveness faded for many. All of the macronutrients are needed by the body to function properly and eating the right protein, fats and carbohydrates in the right proportions is vital to your health (The USDA recommends 18% protein, 29% fat and 53% carbohydrates).

Managing your weight may be challenging, but it is not complex. Simply remember that everything you eat adds calories and that everything you do burns calories. If you eat more calories than you burn, you will put on weight. If you burn more calories that you eat, you will lose weight. Since one pound of body fat equals 3,500 calories, you would need to eat 500 fewer calories than you burn per day in order to lose one pound per week.

Estimating the number of calories you eat every day is fairly easy because food packaging contains calorie information and there are hundreds of websites with calorie listings for every food and portion size imaginable. To estimate the number of calories that you burn daily, multiply your body weight by 15 if you are active or by 13 if you are less active. For example, if you weight 150 pounds and are active, you burn approximately 2,250 calories per day, versus 1,950 calories if you are sedentary (there are also dozens of gadgets and websites to help you estimate the number of calories you burn).

In order to lose weight, you must eat less and get more physical activity. And in order to keep the weight off, your physical activity must roughly equal your calorie intake, habitually. Instead of trying a diet, try building two new habits into your life that you can keep forever:

- Live on Nature's Harvest
- Use Your Body

If you follow the guidelines outlined later in this book for adopting these two habits, you will be able to maintain a healthy weight for the rest of your life.

In a Nutshell: The Carry the Right Weight Rules
1. Know your BMI and manage to it.
2. If you need to reduce your BMI, don't go on a diet. Diets are, by definition, temporary and many are unhealthy.
3. To lose weight and keep it off, *permanently* change your eating habits and your activity habits. To do this, I recommend that you adopt two of the Habits of Healthy People: Live on Nature's Harvest and Use Your Body.
4. In addition, eat smaller portions, eat five times per day to increase your body's metabolism and avoid manufactured foods because they are typically calorie-dense and nutrient-poor.

Chapter 10

Lead an Organic Life

You are what you eat, but you are also what you eat eats.
Michael Pollan

In the fall of 2006, my family and I traveled to be with my father on his horse farm in rural Kentucky. While there, I had the opportunity to visit the cattle farm down the road. My father had been invited by his neighbor to fish on the two ponds on his farm, "any time he wanted." My Dad has never been able to resist the opportunity to drown a worm and he very much liked to teach young children to fish. Battling colon cancer that had metastasized to his spine, liver and lungs, and fearing that he did not have much more time to spend with my children, he insisted that we go fish the ponds despite the recent rain and muddy conditions.

Dad hurried us into the car and loaded every fishing pole he owned and his cooler-size tackle box onto my lap in the front seat. He slowly lowered himself into the driver's seat with a painful grunt and drove the car around the corner and down the road to the cattle farm. The kids chirped with excitement as soon as they heard the crumble of the farm's gravel road. It was as if we had traveled to distant farm country in only three minutes. We rolled along and came to a stop alongside a long white cattle barn that was showing its age. In front of us was a gate that led to the ponds.

Naturally, I would need to open the gate. Dad could not get up and down very easily because of the tumor at the base of his spine. I was, I have to admit, a little irritated at having to extract myself from under the largest fishing tackle box ever made while opening the car door, hoisting eleven fishing poles, and working my feet out of the car into the brackish puddle in front of the gate.

The strong smell of farm animals was in the air, but this was the country, I thought to myself. I splashed over to the gate and noticed a steep hill rising from the gently sloping pasture adjacent to the barn. I eyed the dark, grassless hill as I stood unlocking the gate. It did not appear to be a part of the natural landscape. The car began to pull through the now open gate and I began to realize what was in front of me. I was awestruck at what I was seeing. As alien as it seemed, the brown, grassless hill was a mountain of cow manure the size of a ranch house. As I marveled at the sheer size of this mountain of poo before me, I noticed the grooves the rain had carved in its sides and followed them across the pasture that was gently sloping toward me... All at once, I realized that this city boy was standing shin-deep in a slurry of manure and rain.

"Daddy? Daddy? Daddy!!!" My son was yelling to get my attention as the car rolled past me, but it took a moment to draw my attention away from the enormity of the manure in this place.

"Are those cows dead?"

"What? Where?" I glanced at the noisy cows crowded into the stalls of the barn. As I looked for signs of life in the ones lying down, I noticed that the cows were up to the middle of their bellies in the very same muck slurry of urine, manure and mud in which I stood. How can that be healthy, I wondered?

"No. No, son those cows are alive," I yelled toward the car. "They are just sitting down." I was amazed that the cows literally lived in their own excrement.

As I pushed the gate closed and worked on latching the rusty chain that looked to be as old as the barn, I saw what my son had been asking me about. Six or eight feet from the living cows lay two dead cows with sores all over their bodies and bellies swollen like balloons, their skinny legs stiff and straight. They must have been dragged to this spot to be disposed of, but their location seemed awfully close to the living cows, I thought.

I closed the gate and climbed onto the trunk. There looked to be several more gates before we reached the pond, and the fishing poles and my Dad's gargantuan tackle box made getting in and out of the passenger seat a real treat. The contrast between this place and the farm I had expected was a shock and it began to get to me, I must admit.

As we passed through the second gate and crested the hill, we were among thirty to forty head of cattle, ambling along beside the car. The kids, quickly forgetting about the cows they saw by the barn, now got to see the animals up close. They studied the herd and each child picked out his favorite cow.

My daughter, the animal lover, spotted a calf standing with its mother, "Look – there's a baby," I could hear her say from inside the car. "A baby cow... Awww. He's with his mommy."

The calf was nursing on its mother's udder and didn't release as we approached. As we drove closer to the pair, the mother cow, clearly panicked, straightened its head to look for an escape. As it did, its profile revealed a grotesque, opaque eyeball, surrounded by what looked like maggots and some scarring and scabs. The kids, who had all been focusing on the calf and its mother, let out a collective, "eeeeeeewwwwww!"

I glanced in from my seat atop the trunk of the car and saw my father's reflection in the rear view mirror looking back at me. This was not the quaint farm visit with his grandchildren that he had envisioned. This was a livestock horror show. These cows were sick and dying. Beyond the rear view mirror, I saw our fishing destination: a grimy puddle overgrown with algae.

"Makes me want to get a hamburger," my Dad joked.

Were all modern cattle farms like this, I wondered? I had driven by thousands of cows on car trips, but I drove by at sixty miles per hour. This can't be good for our health, I thought.

The Modern Farm
Before the advent of modern agribusiness, American famers grew multiple crops and had a variety of livestock. This type of farming not only provided for most of the food and income needs of the farmer's family, but it was also biologically necessary. Certain crops helped prepare the soil for other crops to grow – like soybeans for corn – and so farmers would rotate them in the various fields of a farm. As plants died, insects, earthworms and microscopic soil creatures consumed their bodies, excreting waste and releasing nutrients back into the soil, feeding the next generation of plants. Livestock on a traditional farm ate grass, nourished by the sun's energy, and the cow's manure returned the earth's nutrients to the depleted soil in a concentrated form. In addition, natural

predators and parasites helped to keep destructive, plant-eating insects under control.

Following World War II, farming and our food chain dramatically changed. Nitrate, originally mined from the earth, had been used to make ammonium nitrate for explosives for many years. Synthetic nitrogen was first developed by Fritz Haber, a German chemist, during World War I when Germany was cut off from its nitrate mines by its enemies. During WWII, synthetic ammonium nitrate was manufactured in significant quantities in the U.S. using fossil fuels like natural gas and petroleum. When the war ended, however, the U.S. found itself with a surplus of the chemical and was looking for a peacetime use for it. Because it contained a concentrated form of available nitrogen, which is central to the formation of plants but not widely accessible in the earth in the form that plants need, the U.S. Department of Agriculture offered the ammonium nitrate to farmers to put on their crops and synthetic fertilizer was born. (It is also interesting to note that the poisonous gasses used in World War II were the foundation on which the chemical pesticide industry was formed).

When synthetic fertilizers were introduced, farmers were able to grow crops like corn more densely for higher yields and they did not have to worry about rotating crops to nourish the land – synthetic fertilizer would do that. So, farmers began to grow a single crop all year round (this has become known as monoculture). Before synthetic chemicals were used, farmers needed a diversity of crops and animals to support nature's processes – the sun fed the soybeans, the soybeans caused nitrogen to be released in the soil, the nitrogen-rich soil and the sun fed the corn and the grass, the corn and grass fed the farmer and his cattle, and the cattle and the decaying corn plants fertilized the fields. With synthetic chemicals, however, farmers discovered that they could grow the same crops in the same field season after season.

With so much growing capacity, farmers soon found themselves with an excess of synthetically grown corn and they began feeding the corn to the cattle. This mishap proved prosperous for the farmers when they discovered that they could raise cattle more efficiently on trough corn and not have to rotate cattle from field to field when a field's grass was eaten. They also soon learned that cows could reach slaughter weight faster on corn than they could on grass. Before the advent of modern farming techniques, cows would graze on grass and reach slaughter weight (approximately 1,200 pounds) in four or five years. Modern cows, by contrast, are fed a steady diet of genetically modified, chemically-grown corn, fat supplements, protein supplements (which often include the fat of their own species, fish protein, chicken waste, chicken feathers, etc.) and roughage and can now reach slaughter weigh in just over a year.

To ensure that the cows can be monetized, they are also fed enormous amounts of growth hormones and antibiotics. For example, dairy farmers inject their cattle with hormones to increase their annual milk production from 500 pounds to nearly 3,000 pounds. Of the more than 35 million pounds of antibiotics produced per year by pharmaceutical companies, the majority of those antibiotics go to animals. Because cattle farms and feed lots are so full of waste and because cattle typically live in such close quarters, a steady diet of antibiotics is the only thing that keeps them alive.

Every day, modern cows eat approximately 34 pounds of food, turning that into four pounds of meat. Unfortunately for the cow, and, as it turns out, for you and me, the biochemical makeup of the modern cow's diet is not the same as the diet it had evolved to eat. Nature never intended for cattle to subsist on corn, let alone fat and protein supplements, growth hormones and antibiotics. For centuries, cattle have eaten grass nourished by the sun's energy and the earth's balanced ecological processes. Today, instead of converting sunlight into grass into protein, modern cattle farmers convert petrochemicals into corn into protein (the process of creating a 1,200 pound cow consumes approximately 35 gallons of oil) and you and I eat it.

No wonder the cows on the farm I visited looked so sick. They are fed food that they were not intended to eat in quantities they were not intended to eat with toxins and drugs that their bodies cannot degrade and expel. This is done to hang as much marketable meat on the skeletons of these animals as possible, as quickly as possible.

However, this is contrary to nature. Nature is diverse, with many plants and animals living alongside one another in a balanced ecological lifecycle. When you take a natural organism that has evolved over thousands of years on a particular diet and drastically change its diet, feeding it foods than it has ever eaten, feeding it fractions of food dissected industrially and adding synthetic chemicals to make the food production process more efficient, you are going to upset that animal's delicate biological and chemical balance.

Is it possible that cows are degenerating at a molecular level as a result of this shift in their food chain and lifestyle? Is it possible that we are, too? Modern cows and humans are consuming food that they were not intended to eat in quantities they were not intended to eat and are given large amounts of drugs to help maintain their deteriorating health long enough for them to serve society in some way. If someone from 1908 were to walk among a large group of us in 2008, would we look like the degenerating herd of cows to him?

Industrial Agriculture
In order to keep up with growing demand for food in the 1960's and 1970's, the world experienced a revolution and farms, which had already been working on increasing yields, became corporations. Fertilizers, chemicals, hormones, pesticides, herbicides, antibiotics, genetic alterations and more subtle growing changes dramatically improved yields and fed the world. Plants and animals became really big business.

With an industrial revolution in farming came a dramatic revolution in eating (and, probably not coincidentally, health), but most people never knew it. For example, people living in modernized countries today derive a significant portion, and in many cases a majority, of their calories from food grown with synthetic nitrogen. So, instead of deriving their nutrition from the sun's energy, beginning in the 1960's or so, they started to derive their nutrition from fossil fuel energy. The sun-soil combination isn't as productive as synthetic fertilizer. A farmer's yields, and therefore his profits, are larger using synthetic fertilizer. So, instead of converting sunshine into food, farms now convert fossil fuels like petroleum into food.

Consider the tomato. Once a wild plant, tomatoes have become an engineered product of modern industrial agriculture. Year after year, the most desirable seeds have been hand-selected to produce bigger and bigger tomatoes, which – along with heavy doses of fertilizer and pesticides – create the Barry Bonds of tomatoes - huge fruits nearly the size of an infant's head. The next time you are in a store that carries organic produce, compare the size of an organic tomato to its agribusiness cousin. The difference in size is remarkable.

Industrial agriculture continues to evolve and change our food supply. One example is the genetic modification of our food. Genetically modified foods are foods that have been genetically altered, typically to improve crop yields. For example, some genetically modified crops now even produce their own pesticide. While this is cheaper and easier for farmers than spraying pesticide on crops, it introduces new chemical combinations into our bodies that we don't have the science to understand today. Despite the fact that we don't yet understand the health implications of these genetic alterations, the genetically modified food has become incredibly common on store shelves. For instance, 2% of soybeans grown in the U.S. in 1996 were genetically modified, but by 2005, the number had grown to 87%.

Food is now bioengineered by scientists to grow bigger, stay ripe longer, repel insects and transport better (to increase crop yield and, therefore, profit). However, our bodies haven't changed. They still have the same nutritional, biological and chemical requirements they did thousands of years ago. Were it not for the modernization of farming into industrial agriculture, many believe, we simply would not have been able to feed the world's exploding population. However, it certainly makes me wonder if we have used our ingenuity to feed the world's growing population and poisoned it inadvertently. What has four decades of consumption of synthetically-altered food done to the delicately balanced chemistry of the human race?

I believe that time will show that agriculture has been one of the most ill-conceived of modern human endeavors. We eradicate entire ecosystems of plant life to plant fields of a single genetically modified plant, spray it with pesticides, herbicides and chemical fertilizer to produce a harvest of food that is likely unsafe for human consumption. Is it just me or does it seem crazy that the same chemicals that are used to make weapons to kill people (synthetic nitrogen in bombs, neurotoxins in poison gases) are used to grow our food? Should we be surprised if we learn that the same chemicals that kill humans when used in weapons also kill humans when used in farming?

Interestingly, there are also parallels between the earth's environmental problems and our health problems. The fossil fuels that are used to manufacture the synthetic chemicals we use to grow our food pollute the earth and its atmosphere and, one could easily conclude, our bodies. Is a human body degenerated in the same way as our environment? Is our own complex chemistry and biology delicately in balance like the Earth's? Is the Cumulative Effect the health equivalent of global warming? More importantly, are they related?

It is not far fetched to think that the chemicals that are used to make weapons are not good to sprinkle on our food. And it is not far fetched to think that humans and the earth have similar "systems." They have developed together over thousands of years. Although I may be written off as a conspiracy theorist of the highest order, ask yourself how many times per week you hear about the rising cost of health care and the effects of global warming. Maybe they are completely unrelated results of modernization, but then again, maybe they aren't.

Synthetic Food Production

Generally, scientists believe that humans are simply chemical bodies governed by their chemical reactions. This helps to explain the prominence of chemicals (also known as drugs) in medical science. If you believe that people are nothing more than walking chemical reactions, then using chemicals to modify human chemistry seems very logical. However, the inconsistency that really bothers me is that medical science, for the most part, does not acknowledge that the chemicals used in food production (like pesticides, fossil fuels, synthetic fertilizer, hormones, and antibiotics) have an impact on our chemistry too. Why do they think that Merck's and Pfizer's chemicals have an impact on our chemistry but Ortho's and Scotts' chemicals do not? There is enough empirical evidence to carry on for pages about the dangers of the chemicals in our food supply, but rather than write an exhaustive volume here, I will, instead, examine one case in point – pesticides – to increase your awareness of the risks of eating industrially farmed food.

Every year, more than two billion pounds of pesticides are spread in America. Pesticides include insecticides, herbicides and fungicides. We come into contact with pesticides because they are used on nearly all food crops and they are used in yards, parks and recreational areas. In addition, because most modern farm animals graze on pesticide-covered food and fields, the animal products we eat often contain pesticides. This is because pesticides are not easily eliminated from an animal's body and wind up being stored in fat cells.

Most insecticides are designed to attack and destroy the central nervous system of target pests, ultimately killing them. When we consume or come into contact with these pesticides, is it possible that they are attacking our central nervous systems, too? Could that play a part in the rise in Attention Deficit Disorder, Alzheimer's, senility, dementia, Parkinson's, Lou Gehrig's disease and other neural disorders that we are experiencing? Without detailed scientific study and probably about 30 years of scientific advancement, it is difficult to be certain. But it seems likely enough to cause you to think twice about what you feed your family. Consider the following data:

- The EPA has identified 64 pesticides that are potentially carcinogenic (able to cause cancer).
- There appears to be a link between pesticides and breast cancer. Because toxins like pesticides are stored in fatty tissue in the body, when a woman eats meat and whole milk products, the toxins she ingests (from the animal fat) get stored in the fattiest parts of her body – like the breast. It is also interesting to note here that the prostate is a fatty gland in the male body where cancer is becoming increasingly common.
- People with long-term, low-level exposure to pesticides have a 70 percent higher incidence of Parkinson's disease than people who have not been exposed much to bug sprays.
- There is a suspicion that Alzheimer's and dementia are related to chemicals such as pesticides and solvents that cannot be broken down and eliminated from the body and wind up being stored in the body's fatty tissue (like the brain). Alzheimer's affects nearly 5 million people in the U.S. and with an aging population, that figure is set to rise dramatically. It leads cancer as the most feared health problem for today's elderly.

You are a chemical and biological being. You have many complex chemical and biological processes and interactions that take place in your body every second, most of which science and medicine don't understand. When you introduce man-made chemicals into this intricately balanced environment, there will be unintended chemical and biological reactions. When you introduce dozens of man-made chemicals into this intricately balanced environment every day for 40 years (14,600 days), there will inevitably be equally complex consequences that manifest themselves in a number of ways including, very possibly, disease.

What is Organic?

The mainstream availability and acceptance of organic food is a relatively recent phenomenon. Previously only sought out by hardcore twig-eaters, organic food now lines the cupboards of many middle class soccer moms. Organic food sales in the U.S. totaled $13.8 billion in 2005, up from $3.6 billion in 1997, and there were approximately 550,000 acres of certified organic crops grown in the U.S. in 2005, nearly double the amount grown in 1997. But what does organic really mean?

In 1990, the United States Congress passed the Organic Foods Production Act, which directed the United States Department of Agriculture to create a set of regulations for organic agriculture. Finally, in 2002 (twelve *short* years later), the USDA and the National Organics Standards Board passed what is known as The Organic Rule. The following is a summary.

- Organic fruits, vegetables, grains, etc. are grown without the use of genetically engineered seeds, sewage, long-lasting pesticides, herbicides or fungicides.
- Organic meat is from livestock that is free from antibiotics and growth hormones, fed organically-grown feed, and given access to the outdoors.
- Processed food that is organic contains organic ingredients and is free from irradiation, all genetically modified ingredients and synthetic preservatives.
- All foods labeled "organic" must be certified by a USDA-accredited agency.
- Foods labeled "100% organic" must contain only organically grown/produced ingredients excluding salt and water.
- Foods labeled "organic" must contain at least 95% organically grown/produced ingredients. The remainder must be ingredients that the USDA agrees are not available in organic form.
- Foods labeled "made with organic ingredients" must contain at least 70% organically grown/produced ingredients.

It is important to note, however, that the organic rule does not cover food from cloned animals. The FDA has decided that food from cloned animals is safe to eat and does not require special labeling. Consumer groups say labels are a must because surveys have shown people to be uncomfortable with the idea of cloned livestock (64 percent said they were uncomfortable in a 2006 poll by the Pew Initiative on Food and

Biotechnology). However, the FDA concluded that cloned animals are "virtually indistinguishable" from conventional livestock and that no identification is needed to judge their safety for the food supply.

I do not understand the logic in excluding genetically engineered plants and including genetically engineered animals in the organic category. I think the risk is the same – that we are consuming some genetically tweaked food that affects human health in a way that science cannot understand today – but the FDA does not see it that way. Nonetheless, the Department of Agriculture has done a good job, in my opinion, of creating a standard for organic food labeling that does not create enormous loopholes for consumer product companies to sneak through. You can feel very confident when eating foods labeled "100% organic" that you are getting nutrition without potentially harmful synthetic chemicals.

According to the international organic farming organization IFOAM, "The role of organic agriculture, whether in farming, processing, distribution, or consumption, is to sustain and enhance the health of ecosystems and organisms from the smallest in the soil to human beings." Organic farming avoids or largely excludes the use of synthetic chemicals like fertilizers and pesticides, plant growth regulators, and livestock feed additives, all elements common in industrial agriculture. As much as possible, organic farmers rely on crop rotation, crop residues, animal manure and soil cultivation to maintain soil productivity, to supply plant nutrients, and to control weeds, insects and other pests. In addition to its many health benefits, organic farming also:

- Increases the natural productivity of the land
- Reduces toxins in the environment and protects our water resources
- Makes us less reliant on non-renewable fossil fuels (synthetic pesticides and fertilizers are produced using significant amounts of petroleum)
- Preserves the diversity of plants and animals leading to a healthier, more balanced environment

Organic farming is about living within the natural laws of the planet. Our planet has a delicately balanced system with approximately 500,000 plant species and one million species of animals that all integrate into a community of organisms that function as one ecological unit.

However, largely because of industrial agriculture, 30 of the 50,000 edible plant species (.06% of the number of edible plant species) provide 95% of all of the plant calories to the human race and only about 3% of the animal species on the planet are used for meat, milk and muscle. Industrial agriculture's focus on a narrow set of plant and animal species and its intense use of man-made chemicals is upsetting the delicately balanced cycle of nature and setting into motion an ecological breakdown with significant consequences.

Raw Materials
In spite of the obvious benefits of eating and supporting organic agriculture, I often hear people complaining that organic food is too expensive, that organically grown fruits and vegetables are small and discolored, and that organic or "natural" food doesn't taste as good. In reality, the food industry has distorted our perception of food. Most of us alive today grew up on industrial agriculture and processed food so we are accustomed to low cost food, big, shiny produce and explosive taste. It is a little bit like growing up in Los Angeles where everyone looks 26 and has perfect bodies, I think. If a native of Los Angeles left the city for the first time and visited, say, Toledo, Ohio, they would probably think that the people in Toledo were unusually ugly, old-looking, pale, flat-chested and out of shape. The reality, of course, is that the people in Toledo are "natural" and (many of) the people in Los Angeles are, well, synthetic.

The truth is that industrial agriculture and food processing has become so efficient that food is at *unnaturally* low prices. What I mean is that industrially produced food is too cheap to be healthy. The methods used in modern agriculture and modern food production to grow and produce food that can compete in an international commodity marketplace are simply not healthy. Efficiency gains in modern food production, such as the use of synthetic fertilizer and pesticides to increase crop yields, have come at the cost of human health. Unfortunately, those gains have set price expectations in the minds of the consumer that are below the price at which food can be produced naturally.

After years of consistently falling food prices (before the effect of inflation), we have come to expect this cheap food. So, when natural (healthy) farming techniques are used to grow food, and yields of food are at their natural level, farming costs are higher per unit of food – and the prices in the stores reflect that. These are the actual prices, the natural prices, not the synthetically deflated, unnatural ones to which we have become accustomed.

Clearly, certain grocery chains add a higher markup to organic foods because they tend to be preferred by higher income shoppers, but competition always takes care of that. We would all like to spend less money on food, but let's face it; they are the raw materials of the human being. We shouldn't necessarily be looking for the best price on bread, tomatoes, milk, apples and hamburger. We should instead be looking to get the healthiest raw materials that we can afford.

In addition to expecting cheap prices, consumers have become trained to expect food to look a certain way. For example, synthetically grown fruits and vegetables are unnaturally large, but here again our perception has been distorted because we are so accustomed to seeing grapes the size of golf balls. Like professional bodybuilders and baseball players that hit 60 home runs per year, fruits and vegetables only get that size with synthetic help. Organically grown fruits and vegetables are not small – they are the size they were intended to be.

Often consumers can not only feel the difference in their wallets and see the differences with their eyes, they can taste it, too. It's no secret that the food industry uses sensory marketing to attract and retain consumers of its products and that this has distorted our view of what food is suppose to taste, smell and even feel like. All kinds of weird ingredients – sweeteners, binders, fillers, sodium, coloring agents, and taste enhancers – are added to foods during processing in order to make them more appealing to you and me. And, because the modern diet contains so much processed food, we have learned to expect the explosive tastes that have been designed into processed foods. Unfortunately, many of the ingredients added to food to make it more appealing to the senses are very unhealthy.

In reality, you cannot afford the environmental and health consequences of industrial agriculture and modern food processing. Routinely filling your body with synthetic chemicals is a recipe for disease. It's time to get on the organic bandwagon.

Adventures in Eating Organic

Before leaving for a trip to Europe in March of 2006, I received the standard call from my mother. No matter how old we get, our mothers are still our mothers. In addition to the usual stuff – dress warm, call as soon as you get there, don't trust the French – Mom wanted to talk about food, and not in the usual enjoy-the-wonderful-European-food way. She wanted to talk about bird flu and asked me to promise not to eat poultry of any kind while abroad. "Not even eggs or a turkey sandwich, you hear me?"

Bird flu (avian influenza) is an infection from a particular subtype of the Influenza A virus (H5N1) that can cause severe illness in humans who are infected. Currently, this strain is transmitted by contact with infected birds and has been transmitted from one person to another only in a few cases. Wild birds worldwide carry the viruses in their intestines, but usually do not get sick from them. Avian influenza is very contagious among birds, especially domesticated birds like chickens, ducks, and turkeys that live in cramped conditions on farms.

I told her that my wife had made me promise not to eat beef while abroad a year or so earlier because of mad cow disease and joked that my choices were becoming limited. Mad cow disease, officially known as bovine spongiform encephalopathy or BSE, attacks the central nervous system of cows and kills them. The disease is believed to be spread among cows through BSE-infected beef and bone meal that they are fed. The disease has been linked to a brain-wasting disease in humans called Creutzfeldt-Jakob disease.

She replied that I "would just have to eat fish" while overseas. I replied that I limited my consumption of fish because of the mercury in wild fish and pesticides and pollution in farm-raised fish. I went on to explain that the U.S. Food & Drug Administration standards on poultry, beef and fish were among the lowest in the world and suggested that we may have a false sense of security in America. She wondered aloud as we spoke, "What are we left to eat?" After a pause in speech which, for my Mom, is meaningful, I joked that we were all doomed to some kind of mad-cow-bird-flu-mercury-poisoned miserable death. She did not find this to be very funny.

As I have said, agriculture has been a wonderful success and a terrible mistake. Agriculture's mass farming techniques – fertilizers, pesticides, hormones, antibiotics, genetic modification - have increased food yields enough to have kept pace with massive population growth around the world. However, the same mass farming techniques have altered the chemical and biological harmony of our food supply and resulted in a steady deterioration of the chemical and biological harmony of the human race that lives on that food supply. Feeding herbivorous cattle protein-rich meat and bone meal, and especially that of their own species, is highly unnatural. Raising huge numbers of food animals, like chickens or fish, in extremely cramped and dirty conditions and filling them with chemically-tainted food and synthetic medicine is bound to create chemical and biological consequences. Using chemicals that were intended to kill human beings in wartime to grow their food in peace time is a bit unnerving for me. We're messing with our food supply!

It's Not Just In Our Food

Because of the abundance of synthetic chemicals in our modern world, we come into contact with an enormous amount of potentially harmful toxins on a daily basis and it is important to realize that they are not just in our food supply. They can be inhaled in the air you breathe and they can be absorbed through your skin as well. This is very bad news because synthetic chemicals are, quite literally, everywhere. These products can be extremely toxic, yet they are readily available and easily accessible at the local grocery store or home improvement center. The potential health consequences associated with the use of common household products range from eye and throat irritations, headaches, dizziness and nausea to more serious effects such as skin rashes, burns, liver or kidney damage, cancer, birth defects and death. Because these products are easily obtained, we have a false sense of safety when using these products.

In the U.S. alone, as many as 2,000 new chemical compounds are produced each year, most of which are approved by the EPA without testing. For an article in the October 2006 issue of *National Geographic*, author David Ewing Duncan had himself tested for 320 man-made chemicals and found that many of these chemicals were present in varying degrees in his body. To his great surprise, he discovered that he had significantly elevated amounts of chemical toxins – such as flame-retardants and phthalates, substances found in flexible plastic products, nail polish, fishing lures, adhesives, caulk and paint pigments – in his blood. Although the author was not sure how he wound up with such elevated levels of these toxins, it is not likely that these toxins came from his stomach (via food or drink). It is more probable that these elements made it into his body through his lungs or his skin.

With tens of thousands of them in production, it is almost impossible to live a life completely free from contact with synthetic chemicals. However, there are categories of consumer products that are responsible for the introduction of a significant portion of the harmful toxins that wind up in our bodies. Three of the sources of harmful toxins that I believe are most prevalent and most preventable are personal hygiene products, household cleaners and pesticides.

Personal Hygiene Products - Your skin is often referred to as your body's largest organ and when you put something on your skin or expose your skin to air borne chemicals, they can be absorbed right into your blood stream. Most people do not realize that highly toxic materials exist in the common hygiene products that they use on their bodies every day. Harmful chemicals lurk in traditional shampoo, soap, lotion, perfume, deodorant, antiperspirant, toothpaste, shaving cream, cosmetics, hair dyes, hair gels, hair sprays and nail polish. The average woman applies 168 different chemicals from 12 personal hygiene products every day, according to a 2004 study by the Environmental Working Group. Consumer products companies are allowed to include these poisons in our hygiene products because the amount of the chemical used by consumers at one time is below the Food & Drug Administration's legal limits. However, many scientists are now becoming concerned that long-term, low-level exposure to chemicals may be just as dangerous as short-term, high-dose exposures. Below are just a few examples of the chemicals that exist in common personal hygiene products:

- Shampoos commonly contain cresol, formaldehyde, glycols, nitrates/nitrosamines and sulfur compounds. These chemicals are known to cause diarrhea, fainting, dizziness, kidney and liver damage and formaldehyde is a suspected human carcinogen.
- Hair sprays contain butane propellants as well as formaldehyde resins. Butane is an asphyxiant with side effects that range from nausea and vomiting at low doses to hallucinations, coma and sudden death at high doses. As in shampoos above, formaldehyde is a suspected human carcinogen and may contribute to cancer formation.
- Antiperspirants and deodorants commonly contain aerosol propellants, ammonia, formaldehyde, triclosan and aluminum chlorhydrate. You know about formaldehyde from above. Aluminum

is associated with the formation of Alzheimer's disease and senility and triclosan can combine with chlorine in tap water to form chloroform, a probable human carcinogen.

- Skin moisturizers often contain glycols, phenol, fragrance, and artificial colors. These chemicals can cause diarrhea, fainting, dizziness, and kidney and liver damage.

The next time you are in the shower, read the ingredients on the back of your shampoo bottle. The list is one that only a chemist could love. Then imagine taking the top off of your shampoo and drinking it. Not only would it taste awful, you wouldn't want to ingest all of those chemicals into your body, right? Yet, every time you wash your hair you *do* take those unpronounceable chemicals into your blood stream *right through your scalp*. Then consider that you apply a deodorant and possibly an antiperspirant under each arm every day. Antiperspirants block perspiration, a natural process that allows the body to detoxify itself. Ironically, by using a typical deodorant with antiperspirant, you are introducing harmful chemicals into your body and then blocking the exit. It is like setting a fire in a theater and then blocking the doors!

Virtually all of the hygiene and beauty products we use contain fragrances to make them more appealing to our sense of smell. However, the presence of a fragrance in a product, no matter how sweet or natural it smells, can indicate the presence of up to 4,000 separate ingredients, most of which are synthetic. The US National Institute of Occupational Safety and Health evaluated 2,983 fragrance chemicals for health effects in 1989 and they identified 884 of them as toxic substances (roughly 30%). Many compounds in fragrance are human toxins and suspected or proven carcinogens and clinical observations have shown that exposure to fragrances can affect the central nervous system.

Many, if not most, common personal hygiene and beauty products contain harmful chemicals that you should avoid putting onto (and into) your body. The good news is that there are highly effective alternatives for all of these products. By doing a little bit of research or just beginning to shop for your family at stores that carry natural alternatives, you can reduce the amount of harmful chemicals to which you and your family are exposed. I shop at Whole Foods and, in particular, I use natural shampoo, conditioner, body soap, toothpaste and deodorant. I avoid makeup (you will be happy to learn), hair products (have you seen my picture?), shaving cream (I use natural soap) and skin lotion. There are many, many hygiene and beauty products that do not contain harmful chemicals and they are becoming more broadly available. Taking the time to do a little research and experiment with a few different brands of products to find the ones you like is a worthwhile investment. Doing this will significantly reduce the chemical toxins that you are exposed to on a daily basis.

Household Cleaners - Prior to WWII, most household cleaning tasks were accomplished using relatively benign, common household products such as lemon and baking soda. With the increase in production of petroleum-based chemicals following the war, corporations began to manufacture household cleaning products containing specific chemical agents that would target common cleaning challenges. Today, most people are accustomed to buying products that are custom-designed for the many surfaces, materials and rooms in their homes. This shift brought with it a considerable increase in human exposure to harmful synthetic chemicals.

Unfortunately for the common consumer, manufacturers of cleaning products are not compelled by law to list the chemicals used in their products on their packaging. In addition to dozens of neurotoxins and carcinogens in common household cleaning products, some of the most alarming stories revolve around chemicals known as reproductive toxins, which are used in common liquid laundry detergents and toilet cleaners and have recently been declared toxic under the Canadian Environmental Protection Act. Also known as endocrine disrupters, these chemicals are called "gender benders" by environmentalists because they are believed to cause reproductive problems.

Below is a list of some common household cleaning products, the synthetic chemicals they typically contain, and the health risks associated with those synthetic chemicals.
- Air freshener and deodorizers contain formaldehyde and other chemicals. The chemicals in these products are carcinogenic, an irritant to eyes, nose, throat, and skin, and may cause nausea, headaches, nosebleeds, dizziness, memory loss, and shortness of breath.
- Bleach, disinfectants and spot removers contain sodium hypochlorite. They can irritate or burn skin, eyes, respiratory tract and may cause pulmonary edema or vomiting and coma if ingested.

- Drain cleaners and oven cleaners contain sodium or potassium hydroxide. These chemicals can inhibit reflexes, cause burns to skin and eyes, and are poisonous if swallowed. Drain cleaners also contain trichloroethane, which causes liver and kidney damage if ingested.
- Floor cleaner waxes contain diethylene glycol and petroleum solvents. These chemicals can cause central nervous system depression, kidney and liver lesions, and skin and lung cancer.
- Furniture and floor polishes contain petroleum distillates or mineral spirits and nitrobenzene. The chemicals in these products are associated with skin and lung cancer and birth defects, are an irritant to skin, eyes and nose, and entry into lungs may cause pulmonary edema vomiting, and death.
- Toilet bowl cleaners contain sodium acid sulfate or oxalate or hypochloric acid and chlorinated phenols. These chemicals can cause burns from skin contact or inhalation and ingestion may be fatal. In addition, they can cause respiratory, circulatory, or cardiac damage.
- Window cleaners contain diethylene glycol. This chemical can cause central nervous system depression and degenerative lesions in the liver and kidneys.

Contrary to what you see on TV, you do not need a different cleaning product to clean each surface in your home. Multi-purpose cleaners can reduce the number of cleaners you use and reduce the number of hazardous products in your home. In addition, most cleaning chores can be easily handled without any toxic products at all. Everyday ingredients like baking soda, vinegar, salt, lemon juice, vegetable oil, soap, borax, hydrogen peroxide and washing soda can do the job just as well as they did in the old days. Consumer demand and recognition of the hazards of many chemical ingredients are leading more companies to manufacture less toxic cleaning products. Like hygiene and beauty products, you need to do a little shopping around and probably some experimentation with different brands of less toxic cleaners, but the investment of your time is definitely worth the benefits to your health.

Pesticides - Earlier in this chapter, we discussed the array of health risks associated with being exposed to the chemicals in pesticides. Yet it has become customary for people to use pesticides to kill (mostly) harmless insects, plants and plant diseases around their homes. Three out of four U.S. households regularly use pesticides in their home or garden. These homeowners spread approximately 76 million pounds of pesticides around their living spaces each and every year.

To reduce your exposure to toxic chemicals, I recommend that you completely eliminate the use of synthetic pesticides, herbicides and fungicides in and around your home. Now, before you turn the page and write this off as impractical advice, let me say that I have done it myself and it was simple and did not significantly increase the "pest" population in my life. I admit that when I told my wife that we were stopping our home pest control service, she was very apprehensive. She had visions of roaches roaming the kitchen at night and an infestation of ants in our pantry. I was concerned with the thought of eliminating our lawn service because I worried that our lawn would be the eye sore of the neighborhood: patchy grass overrun with weeds and beetles eating all of my shrubs and trees. However, none of this has come to pass. After three years, we have not experienced an infestation of bugs in our home or yard, and our lawn is not overrun with weeds or disease.

I confess that I was conditioned to believe that I needed synthetic chemicals to have a pest-free home and a good looking yard. Clearly, synthetic chemicals can be effective against major pest, weed or fungus problems around the yard and house, but that narrow use has evolved into the idea that we need to broadly and consistently use these chemicals to maintain a pest-free home and yard. This, quite simply, is not the case.

To keep your home pest-free, I found that the best offense is a good defense. The first step is to make the house, especially the kitchen, unattractive to pests by cleaning up food immediately and completely after eating, keeping hard-to-reach areas clean, and removing clutter that can hide pests. Store foods that are attractive to pests – such as flour – in the refrigerator. Also, holes in exterior walls should be closed off and garbage should be kept tightly covered. In addition, a number of nontoxic substances can be used to ward off pests in the event that they do show up in your house. Generally, they contain highly fragrant substances like peppermint, cloves and citrus oil, and can easily be found online or at your local home center or hardware store.

Creating a beautiful lawn and garden without synthetic chemicals is not as hard as you may think, either. Organic lawn and garden care may be more work and more expensive at first, but you will wind up with a lawn that is easier to care for, is safer, and is even more resistant to drought. There are a few very basic guidelines to organic lawn care:

- Mow high and leave the clippings. Mow your lawn at 2.5 to 3 inches in height to deter weeds. Don't bag the clippings as they provide excellent nutrition for the soil as they decompose.
- Use organic fertilizers. Non-synthetic, organic fertilizers can be found in garden centers and most home improvement chains.
- Use organic herbicides (weed killers). Organic herbicides such as organic corn gluten are widely available. They do not act as fast or as completely as herbicides made with synthetic chemicals, but they are far safer. Under no circumstances should you treat your entire lawn for weeds. Whether you use synthetic or organic herbicides, you only need to spot-treat the areas where weeds are present.
- Use non-toxic pesticides (bug killers). In hardware stores, look for brands of safer insecticides that use soap-and water solutions.

With over 70,000 synthetic chemicals in production, it probably comes as no surprise to you to learn that most pesticides contain chemicals that are very toxic. Simply pick up your roach spray, lawn fertilizer, mosquito repellent, weed killer, etc. and read the label. Once you've read the label (the ingredient list, the warnings, and the "in the event of" medical advice), consider whether the chemicals in this product are safe for you to put into your body. I think you will agree that eliminating dangerous pesticides from your home and yard and seeking out natural alternatives is a worthy investment in your health.

Leading an Organic Life
World War II ushered in an era of war-related chemical research, and when the war ended, factories that produced chemicals for killing the enemy (ironically) became factories that produced chemicals for simplifying our lives. Today, we live in an increasingly toxic world as a result of the chemical revolution. Toxins enter our bodies through the air we breathe, the water we drink, the foods we eat, the products we use to clean and beautify our bodies, the medicines we take and the consumer products we use at home and at work. With an understanding of the Cumulative Effect, you can begin to comprehend how these toxins can degenerate the cells and tissues of the human body, leading to many of the diseases that are now reaching epidemic levels in our population.

It is really hard for any unbiased, rational person to deny the link between the many degenerative conditions that have grown to epidemic proportions and the synthetic chemicals that have grown exponentially in unison. In order to live a healthy life in this type of an environment, it is critical that you vigilantly strive to reduce the amount of toxins that enter your body. Get into the habit of paying attention to what you eat, what you drink, what you breathe, what you use for hygiene and beauty, and what products you use around the house. This type of preventative focus is a critical element to avoiding The Cumulative Effect.

If you simply pay attention, I estimate that you can easily reduce the synthetic chemicals that enter your body by 50%. If you are really vigilant, you can probably reduce the synthetic chemicals that enter your body by 70% - 80%. Unfortunately, without really disrupting your lifestyle (and probably living in a bubble), I do not think that you can ever reduce your exposure to toxic chemicals by much more than that. The 70,000 synthetic chemicals produced around the world have become absolutely pervasive in our lives and it is virtually impossible to escape them, especially in the air we breathe. As a result, it is critical that you also take steps (as outlined in other chapters of this book) to eliminate the toxins that do enter your body as efficiently as possible.

While synthetic chemicals are composed of the same atoms and molecules that make up all matter on earth, these man-made chemicals are different from anything that exists in nature and we do not know all the issues that surround their use in our environment and in our bodies. If you are concerned about your health, I think that you will conclude, as I have, that you should be very thoughtful about the synthetic chemical containing products that you buy and use. Making simple choices can dramatically reduce the number and amount of synthetic chemicals that you come into contact with on a daily basis.

In a Nutshell: The Lead an Organic Life Rules
1. Consume only certified organic meat and dairy. This means selecting meat and dairy products that are from animals that are free from antibiotics and growth hormones, fed organically-grown feed, and given access to the outdoors for their entire life.
2. Consume organic fruits, vegetables, grains and nuts. If you cannot find or afford organics, make sure that you are thoroughly cleaning your produce before you eat it with a fruit and vegetable wash.

3. Use organic personal hygiene products. Start by replacing your shampoo, conditioner, soap, body lotion, shaving cream, cosmetics and especially your deodorant.
4. Use natural household cleaning products. There are an abundance of natural alternatives to these products that are effective multi-purpose cleaners for your house.
5. Stop using pesticides. These nerve toxins disable and kill insects and household pests and no one can say with certainty what they do to your nervous system and those of your children when used inside your home and in your yard.

Chapter 11

Detox Your Body

Sickness is the vengeance of nature for the violation of her laws.
Charles Simmons

If you live in a developed country, your body is probably under assault by a continuously increasing load of toxins. We have polluted our world to such an extent that we are becoming polluted, too. Just think about our air, our water and our food – the three basic necessities for supporting human life. Our air is toxic, our water is polluted and our food contains poisonous chemicals.

Every day, we inhale roughly 35 pounds of air in 20,000 breaths. Unfortunately, that air is polluted by exhaust from cars, busses and airplanes, industrial air pollution and more. Carbon monoxide, emitted when fuel is burned, makes up the majority of our air pollution. Heavy metals, emitted from waste incineration, smelting and oil refining, make up a substantial portion as well. And indoor air pollution is just as bad. In fact, the air inside a new home can be five to 20 times more polluted than the air outside. Just taking a breath can be harmful to your health.

As discussed in detail earlier in the book, our drinking water supply can be quite dangerous to our health. Our water is tainted with pesticides, fertilizer, industrial chemicals, industrial waste and lead and then we add some other potentially harmful chemicals in the water "treatment" process for good measure (chlorine and fluoride). Water, although an abundant natural resource, is finite and becomes increasingly polluted as the earth's population grows.

As covered in an earlier chapter, every year, nearly two billion pounds of pesticides are sprayed on crops grown in the U.S. That is more than seven pounds of pesticide for every man, woman and child living in America. The Environmental Protection Agency has identified more than 50 cancer-causing pesticides in use today and, although the EPA has moved to ban some of the most harmful substances, manufacturers are still able to export them for use in countries that import food right back to us. In addition, our supply of beef, pork and poultry is tainted with hormones, antibiotics and pesticides and much of the fish we eat is polluted from chemical run off or grown in waste-polluted fish farms.

Simply breathing, drinking and eating can lead to a build up of synthetic chemicals, toxins and even your body's own metabolic waste in the cells, tissues and organs of the body. It is estimated that there are approximately one hundred trillion cells (100,000,000,000,000) in your body and each one of them probably has a build up of accumulated waste, reducing their efficiency and, quite literally, slowing you down. When cells are clogged with waste, they are not able to perform their functions normally and this causes you to become lethargic and lack energy. In addition, this build up can severely affect the operation of those organs and tissues. Often, these buildups aren't severe enough to be recognized as diseases unto themselves, but they can lead to quite a few problems throughout the body and may contribute to the eventual formation of disease.

The body has a difficult time eliminating many of these toxins and, as a result, they either get recirculated into the bloodstream, wreaking havoc throughout the body, or they get stored in the liver, body fat or other tissues and organs of the body. The human body is a delicately balanced biological and chemical entity. When you add dozens of synthetic chemicals into the body, unintended "reactions" can occur and, if those chemicals persist in the body, they can alter the fundamental chemistry of a system, organ or the whole body. Common changes include pH imbalances, imbalances in bacteria and fungus and cell or DNA damage.

The human body has a tremendous ability to withstand the intake of toxins and cleanse itself, but over time, the enormous amount of toxins that the average person comes into contact with in a developed country eventually overwhelms the body's defenses. Toxins then build up in the body and can have a degenerating effect on tissue and cells, leading to sickness and, eventually, disease. In fact, this may very well be the cause of the incredible rise of many chronic health problems with unknown causes such as migraine headache, ALS/ Lou Gehrig's Disease, Parkinson's Disease, Alzheimer's, Attention Deficit Disorder, etc. This is a grim thought, considering the abundance of synthetic chemicals in use today.

Of course, there is a silver lining in this dark cloud. These toxic buildups can be removed and purged when you Detox Your Body. Detoxification comes in many forms and refers to many different programs that cleanse the body of toxins. While there are many detoxification programs available, they differ in their actions and their intent.

Detoxification may refer generically to the purification of the body through *everyday detoxification routines* or more specifically to the *cleansing* of the body's cells and the systems that your body uses to detoxify itself. Everyday detoxification routines are practices that, if done habitually, help to reduce the toxins stored in the body over time. Everyday detoxification routines that can help to purify the body's cells include a diet high in phytochemicals, antioxidants, fiber and water; frequent vigorous exercise; effective skin care and deep breathing exercises.

Cleansing, on the other hand, refers to temporary detoxification programs that are designed to purge your body of built up toxins in a short period of time. These cleansing programs can target the whole body or focus on the liver, kidneys, lungs or bowels since these are the systems that your body uses when it breaks down and eliminates toxins. (The liver is responsible for breaking toxins down into compounds that the body can safely handle and eliminates them through the kidneys as urine, the skin as sweat, the lungs as expelled air and the bowels as feces.) In addition, cleansing programs typically help to clean the blood since the blood carries toxins as waste products.

Effectively detoxifying your body of the build up of toxic substances requires a foundation of everyday detoxification routines supplemented with periodic cleansing. While everyday detoxification routines alone can result in the gradual removal of toxic substances from the body, the detoxification can be slower than the intake of toxins in our chemically abundant lives. When you take in more toxins than you eliminate, an accumulation of toxins will still occur, albeit more slowly than if you did not follow everyday detoxification routines at all.

Therefore, for most people, I recommend a foundation of everyday detoxification routines and annual cleansing. If you work with dangerous chemicals in your job (house cleaning, lawn service, painting, furniture manufacturing, carpet manufacturing, etc.) or you use prescription pharmaceuticals on a regular basis, your intake of toxins is likely higher than average and you need to expel them from your body more often. If this describes you, you may need to increase your cleansing frequency.

Below, I outline the basics of everyday detoxification routines and cleansing programs. Because this book is not intended to give the reader an exhaustive review of any one habit of health, you should seek out additional information on detoxification if you think you may have a particularly acute build up of toxins in one area, such as your liver, to augment your knowledge. There is abundant information available on detoxification online, in bookstores and in health food stores.

Everyday Detoxification Routines
Follow a diet built around nature's harvest. A diet built around nature's harvest (as described earlier in the book) is the foundation of any detoxification program. This type of diet contains the proper amounts of vitamins that feed and nourish the bowels and the liver, as well as other eliminative organs. It includes a valuable source of enzymes and generally does not include foods that cause problems with digestion and elimination such as sugar and processed foods. However, more than anything else, a diet built around nature's harvest includes ample fiber for stimulating elimination of waste from the body.

Fiber in the diet serves two important purposes as it relates to detoxification: it helps to maintain bowel movement regularity and it binds to toxins in the intestines and prevents them from being reabsorbed into the body. The body's filter, the liver, removes toxins from the blood. The bile from the liver carries the toxins out through the bile ducts into the small intestine, through the GI tract and into the colon. In the GI tract, fiber will bind with these toxins, preventing their re-absorption through the intestinal walls. However, if you do not have enough fiber in your diet or if your bowels are not functioning correctly, these toxins can be reabsorbed through the intestinal walls into the body.

Diets rich in red meat and fat and low in fiber are associated with the formation of colorectal cancers. Although genetic factors also influence the risk of colorectal cancer, some studies suggest that adopting a diet low in fat and high in fiber may reduce the risk of colon cancer by as much as 40 percent. The lowest incidence of colon cancer is found in countries where there is a higher intake of fruits and vegetables. These include countries in Africa, Asia and South America where (ironically) poverty prohibits the consumption of large amounts of meat.

Don Colbert, M.D. believes that Americans have a high rate of colorectal cancer "because the foods we eat contain toxins that stay in our gastrointestinal tracts for days simply because we don't get enough fiber in our foods. Because of the lack of sufficient fiber to help with elimination, toxins remain in our gastrointestinal tract and begin to form carcinogens. Eventually, these carcinogens begin to change the cells of the colon." Dr. Colbert goes on to say, "The solution lies in eating fruits and vegetables that contain enough fiber to help bind toxins and eliminate them from the colon."

Many sources recommend that you strive to eat 20 or more grams of fiber every day. Because we are so over-burdened with toxins, I believe that we need more like 30 to 40 grams of fiber daily. However, I am not one that believes in counting nutrients. It is impractical, in my opinion. Instead, focus on building your diet around nature's harvest – fresh fruits and vegetables, whole grains, nuts, seeds, beans and legumes – and make sure that you emphasize the best sources of fiber: beans, whole grains, apples, pears, berries, peas, celery and carrots.

It is important to note here that eating plenty of fiber needs to be complimented with drinking an adequate supply of clean water. Your body needs both water and fiber to move waste through the digestive track efficiently. For more on adequate water consumption, read the chapter Drink from the Fountain of Health.

Keep "it" moving. Not surprisingly, having regular bowel movements is important to detoxification. As discussed above, the liver is the organ that breaks down toxins, but the intestines are primarily responsible for removing most of them from the body. When you don't eliminate the digested food in your colon, toxins that your body has worked so hard to process sit in your colon, get reabsorbed back into your body and poison you.

In his ground breaking book, *The Maker's Diet,* Jordan Rubin said, "The colon is the number one repository for oxidative stress in the body. We hear a great deal in the media about antioxidants and the danger of free radicals, but very few of us realize most of the free radical or oxidative damage is generated in the colon during the final stages of the digestive process! This explains why it is good to eliminate waste often rather than have it languish for days in the digestive tract, generating potentially harmful toxins all the while."

Unfortunately, constipation and irregular bowel movements allow this to happen all too often in populations of modernized countries. I am convinced that this is how my father and so many other men and women wound up with colorectal cancer. My Dad's diet consisted of primarily meat, sweets, refined flour and processed/packaged food. In my lifetime, I don't recall seeing him eat a piece of raw fruit, although he had two dozen fruit trees on his farm. People on high fiber diets that eat a lot of fresh fruit and vegetables can digest their food and have a bowel movement in half the time that it takes people on a diet consisting primarily of meat/refined flour/sugar. That means that fruit, vegetables and grains are not only more nutritious, they help the body eliminate toxins more efficiently.

It is said that you should have a bowel movement for every meal that you eat per day. The average meal takes about four hours to digest so, depending on what time you eat dinner, you should have two to three bowel movements per day. I consider myself pretty darn healthy now and I rarely have three bowel movements per day. I typically have (wow, I can't believe that I am actually writing this) two per day. You should have at least one per day. Any less is unhealthy.

As discussed above, the easiest way to get the bowels moving is a high fiber diet consisting of fresh fruits and vegetables. The extra fiber adds to the bulk of the stool and decreases the bowel transit time, which means better toxin elimination and better health. If you are constipated or have irregular bowel movements, make sure that you are getting 30 – 40 grams of fiber in your diet every day and consuming enough water. If you simply have a high fiber cereal and fruit for breakfast and you drink 64 ounces of water per day, you will be amazed at how "things" improve. In addition, exercise stimulates the colon and regular exercise will regularly stimulate you (see how all of these habits hang together?)

I have also found that the digestion and elimination process works better on a set schedule. If you have a routine (which I highly recommend to support your healthy habits), you will be able to set your watch by your visits to the restroom. I have noticed, by contrast, when I adjust my schedule, particularly when I travel abroad, I have all kinds of issues. When my body thinks its time to be asleep, I am eating, and when it thinks it is time to eat, I am sleeping. In response, my intestines just go on strike. They implement a work slow down until I get home and back on my normal routine and then everything goes back to normal.

If you are experiencing irregular bowel movements despite a healthy diet and consistent schedule, you may need a natural bowel stimulant or laxative. There are many highly effective natural products available to get your bowels moving and they range from the mild (slippery elm) to the moderate (cascara sagrada) to the explosive (aloes and senna). Herbal bowel formulas are excellent because they stimulate the bowel to move and provide it with the nourishment it needs to move on its own. However, one should not become overly dependent on laxatives and bowel stimulants since they deplete potassium and may be addicting. A natural, high fiber diet should be enough to keep your bowels working properly.

Get your antioxidants. Normally, molecules in your body have a positively charged neutron surrounded by negatively charged electrons. Cellular oxidation happens as a function of our normal metabolism, but it can be driven out of control by stress or the intake of second hand smoke, pollution, alcohol, toxins like pesticides or the wrong foods. The high energy radiation from these toxins can attract negatively charged electrons away from their molecules causing those molecules to become unstable. The electrons that have been pulled away from the molecule then seek out another molecule causing the new host molecule to become unstable.

These free radicals damage your cells, tissues and organs as they tear through your body looking for an opposing charge with which to pair up. Oxidative stress is thought to contribute to the development of a wide range of diseases including Alzheimer's disease, Parkinson's disease, rheumatoid arthritis and neurodegeneration in motor neuron diseases. In addition, oxidation is thought to be the primary cause of aging in both the body and the brain.

Antioxidants help your cells to neutralize free radicals that can cause mutations and cellular damage. Antioxidants can pair up with the free electrons, neutralizing them and making the free radical cells once again stable. Antioxidants are naturally occurring phytonutrients found in certain fruits and vegetables, foods, etc. They have been proven over and over again to protect human cells from oxidative free-radical damage. As you know well by now, I recommend that you regularly consume a variety of fruits, vegetables, nuts, seeds, grains and legumes. In addition to being high in fiber, vitamins, minerals and phytonutrients, these foods also contain a good supply of antioxidants. Foods that are high in antioxidants include apples, raisins, blackberries, blueberries, cranberries, prunes, oranges, pink grapefruit, grapes, kiwi, artichokes, spinach, kale, Brussels sprouts, broccoli, beets, red peppers, carrots, tomatoes, beans, pecans, and cinnamon.

Because many people don't typically consume enough fruits, vegetables, nuts, seeds, grains and legumes to combat the oxidative stress occurring in their bodies, taking an antioxidant supplement that contains Vitamins A, C and E could be a wise choice (you may consider taking an antioxidant vitamin supplement that also includes grape seed extract and green tea, as both are significantly more powerful antioxidants than vitamins A and E). Taken correctly, a supplement can supply your body with antioxidants to quench the excess of free radicals that happen as a function of our fast-paced, stress-filled, synthetic lives. If you do supplement your diet with antioxidants, remember that they are not a substitute for a healthy diet; they are supplements, or additions to, a healthy diet. I also recommend that you choose a food-based antioxidant supplement formula rather than the synthetic versions or the individual vitamins and combine them. This helps to ensure that you get the right combinations of vitamins and other active ingredients.

Take care of your skin. It is often said that the skin is the body's largest organ because it covers 17,000 square centimeters of the body. It is also the only organ in the body that interfaces with the outside world and it is used by the body for excreting toxins and waste. It has been documented that our skin's sweat glands, when combined, can perform as much detoxification as both kidneys. Therefore, it is very important to take care of your skin.

It all starts with effective, natural skin care. As discussed in the previous chapter, using synthetic personal hygiene and skin care products is not wise. The chemicals contained in these products are absorbed through our skin into the body and provide more toxins for our liver to deal with. In addition, the use of the wrong type of personal hygiene products or an overuse of skin care products can clog or damage the pores of the skin, preventing the body from sweating effectively, which is a key to eliminating the toxins circulating in the body.

Taking care of our skin is rather simple, it turns out. We need to bathe using natural soaps and care for the skin using only natural oils and products of natural origin. This natural skin care approach should be supported by good nutrition. Since our skin is mainly fat, we need high quality fats and oil from natural sources to give our skin the nutrition it needs.

However, despite your best efforts to care for your body's largest organ properly, your skin's pores often get clogged with dirt or dead skin and the body cannot excrete waste as effectively, trapping toxins inside the body. Exfoliation is a method of cleaning your skin by brushing or scrubbing it. Dry skin brushing helps in removing the outer dead skin layers and keeps the pores open. Exfoliating all of your skin, even in those hard to reach places, is important to maintaining the body's ability to excrete toxins.

I recommend that you exfoliate all of the skin on your body using a soft brush or loofah at least twice per week. While you are dry, vigorously brush all of your skin from your face, neck, shoulders, back, chest, arms – all the way down to the soles of your feet – and then gently rinse off with warm water to wash away the dead skin. I find it most convenient to exfoliate this way while I am in the shower before I turn on the water (you might want to get the water warm before you get in). Another good method of skin brushing is with vigorous toweling off after bathing. Towel roughly until the skin is slightly red. Change towels often because they will contain toxins.

Once your skin is cared for naturally and properly exfoliated, your body is more able to sweat out the toxins that you inevitably consume in your daily life. Perspiration helps the body rid itself of toxins by releasing water through the pores of the skin. The water excreted through your pores carries with it waste products and toxins such as heavy metals.

Regular vigorous exercise virtually guarantees ample perspiration for detoxifying the body. However, if you do not get regular vigorous exercise that causes you to perspire, a sauna is a great alternative. Saunas have been used throughout the world for many, many years because of their ability to improver overall health. The heat in a sauna causes perspiration without vigorous exercise. According to Dr. Colbert, "a sauna stimulates the cellular metabolism and breaks up the water molecules that hold toxins within the body, thus allowing the body to void these toxins through perspiration." Be careful of steam rooms, though. The steam in the steam room is often from unfiltered water and you wind up breathing in dozens of toxic chemicals from the steam while you sweat.

The accumulation of toxins in our bodies in this day and age is unavoidable. In 2005, the Centers for Disease Control released its *Third National Report on Human Exposure to Environmental Chemicals* and it stated that trace elements of industrial chemicals were found in the bodies of all 2,400 people that it randomly tested. Your skin plays an important role in ridding your body of those accumulated toxins. If you take care of your skin through natural skin care and exfoliation and you regularly perspire, your skin will assist in the detoxification of your body and keep you healthy and vigorous.

Breathe deeply. Oxygen is the most vital nutrient for our bodies. It is essential for the integrity of the brain, nerves, glands and internal organs. We can do without food for weeks and without water for days, but without oxygen, we will die within a few minutes. And, as you will learn below, proper breathing can also detoxify your body.

Your body's cells depend on a system known as the lymphatic system to drain off toxic materials. The lymph moves throughout the body by a series of channels, valves and filters (or lymph nodes) and eventually drains into the blood through two ducts located at the base of the neck. These ducts empty the lymph into the veins, which returns it to the liver to be broken down.

When the lymphatic system is working properly, toxins are removed from cells and broken down by the liver. However, when the lymphatic system backs up, cellular waste accumulates in the body, which causes two problems. First, the toxic load on the body increases and unintended chemical reactions in the body can occur. Second, the immune system becomes impaired.

In addition to being part of the body's plumbing and repair system, the lymphatic system is an essential part of the immune system. The lymph nodes also produce substances which fight off invading bacteria and viruses and destroy abnormal cells which develop within the body, such as cancer cells. When there is a backup in the lymphatic system, the immune system is not able to do its job of protecting the body against foreign elements as effectively. As discussed throughout this book, the combination of an increased toxic load and an impaired immune system are two of the primary ingredients of the Cumulative Effect, the leading cause of chronic illness and disease, in my opinion.

Keeping the lymph moving throughout the body can be as easy as breathing deeply. Unlike the cardiovascular system, the lymphatic system lacks any central heart-like organ to pump lymph throughout the lymph vessels. So, gravity, the movement of muscles and simple breathing does the work. And, the more deeply you breathe, the more effectively you move lymph. For example, if you take a deep breath and exhale fully, you're massaging the thoracic duct in the neck upward so that the fluid flows abundantly. In addition, deep breaths expand the lungs and move the organs inside your rib cage gently massaging the lymphatic system.

Exercising moves lymph too, but I am convinced that we are not as active as we need to be to keep the lymph moving consistently. So, a deep breathing habit is an important supplement to the daily activity habit described in the chapter Use Your Body above. There are a wide variety of simple breathing exercises and the best news is that they don't require a lot of effort or time. As an added bonus, breathing exercises are very relaxing, which, as you will learn in the next chapter, is also very important to health.

My favorite breathing exercise is called "The 578" and it is very simple. To do The 578, breathe in through your nose for five seconds, hold that breath deep in your lungs for seven seconds, then exhale through your mouth for eight seconds and repeat. The exhale is done with pursed lips (like you are blowing a kiss) and with the tip of your tongue pressed against roof of your mouth at the ridge just behind your front teeth. Simply count in your head – one, two, three, four, five – as you inhale, hold and exhale. I recommend that you do this 578 cycle 10 times once or twice per day, which takes only three and a half minutes each time, or find another breathing exercise to do for three to ten minutes every day.

I like to do breathing exercises in the car on the way to and from work. The car is a quiet, easy place to do deep breathing exercises and, because I commute twice per day, the car provides a reinforcing framework for the habit. I know the patches of road where I do my breathing exercises and I almost subconsciously start and stop them at the right places. Deep breathing really does make you feel very good and very relaxed, and we could all use a little pick-me-up when we're sitting in traffic. Do The 578 exercise or any other deep breathing exercise once or twice per day and you are well on your way to a productive lymphatic system that rids the body of toxins.

Cleansing

Go fast. Your cells are like tiny sponges. They absorb what you breathe, eat, drink and apply to your skin. And, according to Dr. Don Colbert, your body's pH balance is what determines whether your cells will retain what they absorb or expel them. It turns out that when your body is too acidic, your cell walls become less permeable and cellular waste products cannot be excreted efficiently. "When this occurs," he says, "the mitochondria or energy-producing structures in the cell do not function properly and you usually feel fatigued... free-radical activity increases and the toxic overload just continues to build until your body begins to deteriorate and degenerative diseases occur."

To counter this, Dr. Colbert, and many others in the field of preventative health, recommend fasting. Fasting is a thousands-year old practice used by people throughout history to achieve spiritual clarity. Many biblical figures including Jesus himself fasted for as long as 40 days during times of spiritual exploration and crisis. In recent years, it has been discovered that fasting not only helps to purify the mind and spirit, but it can also purify the body. Since fasting has never been taught in any of America's 127 medical schools, conventional doctors - schooled to deal primarily with symptoms - hold a dim view of fasting. In fact, most traditional doctors appear never to have known, or seem to have forgotten, that all three Fathers of Western Medicine practiced and prescribed prolonged fasting - Hippocrates, Galen and Paracelsus, who declared fasting "the greatest remedy, the physician within."

During fasting, two important things happen to your body. First, your body's pH becomes more alkaline, increasing the permeability of the cell walls, allowing them to excrete cellular waste and accumulated toxins. Second, because you are not taking in solid food, your body begins to autolyze or self-digest, its most inferior and impure materials and metabolic wastes. Dr. Joel Fuhrman, author of *Fasting and Eating for Health*, notes, "The fast does not merely detoxify; it also breaks down superfluous tissue – fat, abnormal cells, plaque and tumors – and releases diseased tissues and their cellular products into the circulation for elimination. Toxic or unwanted materials circulate in our bloodstream and lymphatic tissues and are deposited in and released from our fat stores and other tissues. An important element of fasting detoxification is mobilizing the toxins from their storage areas."

Fasting can take on many forms, but the two dominant types of fasts are water-only fasts and juice fasts. Water-only fasts are severe and can be dangerous so they have become less common. I, Dr. Colbert, and most others recommend short duration juice fasts - one to three day fasts where all you consume are freshly juiced organic fruits and vegetables and filtered water. Both water fasting and juice fasting enable the body's pH to become alkaline and the cells to detoxify themselves and both cause the body to autolyze, yet juice fasting is less severe and less dangerous than water fasting. The many fruit and vegetable juices consumed during a juice fast supply energy, minerals, vitamins, live enzymes, and other nutrients needed by your body during the fast. They also supply the 400 calories or so that is your minimal fuel requirement. Without that minimum caloric intake, your body begins to break-down protein structures to get its fuel.

Proponents of juice fasting believe that the detoxification that occurs helps to increase energy, enhance mental clarity, improve skin appearance, eliminate food allergies, reduce the persistent stress and burden on the digestive system and prevent chronic diseases. Although juice fasts require some planning and discipline, their ability to quickly rid the body of accumulated toxins make them well worth the effort. An unsupervised juice fast can last one to three days (any longer and you will need to be under the supervision of a doctor). To fight the accumulation of toxins in our synthetic lives, I recommend a two-day juice fast done once or twice per year.

To do a juice fast, it is recommended that you begin cleaning up your diet and habits at least a week before the fast. During this preparation period, your diet should consist primarily of organic fruits, vegetables, beans and 64 to 96 ounces of pure, filtered water per day. Alcohol, caffeine, nicotine, refined sugar, dairy, meat, fish, and eggs should be reduced or eliminated from the diet.

During the juice fast itself, you will consume approximately 64 ounces of freshly juiced, organic fruit and vegetable juice per day. All the essential nutrients in fruits and vegetables are locked within their fibers and when they are juiced, these essential nutrients are freed from the fiber and can be absorbed and used directly, requiring a minimum amount of digestive effort. The metabolic energy that would have been used on digestion of solid foods is instead used for cleansing waste and toxins from your body's tissues. Typically, a variety of fruits and vegetables are juiced four or five times per day, enabling you to sip nutrient-rich juice throughout the day. In addition to drinking the juice, you will drink 64 to 96 ounces (depending on your weight) of clean, room temperature water spread throughout the day. Other than the juice and the filtered water, nothing else is consumed during a juice fast.

If you buy your juice commercially, it should be fresh, organic, 100% fruit or vegetable juices and should be pasteurized to eliminate harmful microorganisms. Or, to save money, you can juice your own fruits and vegetables. There are loads of juicer types and models to choose from on the market today. Do a little research on the Internet before buying a juicer. A good place to start is www.discountjuicers.com/compare.html. This site provides a very good education about juicers and a comparison of a broad range of juicer types, models and price points. (I have no affiliation with this company.)

I recommend that you get a combination of organic fruit and vegetable juices during your fast to ensure that you are still getting a variety of nutrients. Typical juicing fruits include apple, peach, pear, mango, blueberry, cherry strawberry, pineapple, nectarine, and cranberry (citrus fruits are avoided because of their acidity). Typical juicing vegetables include carrot, tomato, celery, cucumber, kale, broccoli, cabbage, green pepper, romaine lettuce, spinach, beet, and greens.

It should be noted that when you fast, you may feel a little worse initially. This is referred to as a "healing crisis" and it is a result of your body detoxifying itself. Your energy levels may drop and you may experience a feeling of sickness – nausea, headache, etc. Other common experiences are thickening in the tongue coating, bad breath, unpleasant taste in the mouth, foul-smelling stools, digestive upset, acne, energy fluctuations, mucus in the stools, sinus congestion, skin eruptions, fever, muscle aches or tightness, and gas. The duration of this feeling depends on the length of your detoxification and the extent of your toxicity. Generally, a health crisis only lasts 24 to 48 hours and should be viewed as a good thing because the body is detoxifying itself.

More severe side effects can include fainting, dizziness, low blood pressure, heart arrhythmias, weight loss, hunger, vomiting, diarrhea and kidney problems. If these side effects occur, the fast should be discontinued immediately and it should prompt an immediate visit to a qualified health professional. Pregnant or nursing women and children should not try a juice fast. People with terminal illness, cancer, epilepsy, diabetes, ulcerative colitis, kidney disease, liver disease, anemia, gout, asthma, low blood sugar, eating disorders, nutritional deficiency, underweight, addictions, impaired immune function, infection, low blood pressure, or other chronic conditions should only fast under strict medical supervision. People should not try juice fasts before or after surgical procedures. Fasting can reduce blood proteins and change the way prescription drugs react in the body. If you have health concerns, consult a qualified your health professional before trying a juice fast.

With that said, I am a big proponent of juice fasts and juicing in general because it allows people to get more fruit and vegetable nutrition in their diet. If you want to learn more about juicing or juice fasting, I recommend that you search the Internet. There are a ton of useful, free resources.

Try herbs. Everyday detoxification routines are a good foundation for protecting the body against toxic build up, and periodic fasting helps to cleanse the tissues, lymph and blood of stored waste. However, there are circumstances when the detoxification organs of the body – the liver, kidneys, lungs and intestines – need additional cleansing and repair. In these cases, herbs help detoxification to be organ-specific.
Herbs are foods and they may be combined in varying ways to aid specific organs. For example, the herb milk thistle is best known as a liver tonic. The active ingredient is silymarin, which is reputed to repair liver damage due to alcohol, drugs, hepatitis, and exposure to toxins. Yarrow, another common herb, acts as a blood cleanser and opens the pores to permit free perspiration for elimination of waste, relieving the kidneys. Psyllium husk, yet another common herb, is used to cleanse and lubricate the intestines and colon.

While herbs may be taken at any time for detoxification, they are best when they are used in combination with healthy habits. It does not make any sense to take herbs to cleanse the liver if you drink five beers every night. And, while juice fasts are effective by themselves, they may be reinforced and sped up with herbs, which stimulate the eliminative organs. To learn more about detoxifying herbs, I suggest that you do some research on the Internet, at your local health food store or with a naturopathic health professional.

Detox-ing Your Body
The foundation of everyday detoxification is a healthy diet built around nature's harvest – organic fruits, vegetables, grains, nuts, beans and legumes. Other everyday detoxification routines include maintaining proper bowel function and frequency, taking antioxidants, caring for your skin properly and deep breathing to stimulate the lymphatic system. On top of the everyday detoxification routines, I recommend periodic cleansing via short duration juice fasts. Last but not least, detoxifying herbs can be used to target specific organs of the body that may become overloaded with toxins such as the liver and kidneys.

While a detoxification habit can go a long way toward restoring your health, it is important to remember that it is not a license to live an unhealthy lifestyle. There is no cure-all that gives you the freedom to smoke, drink alcohol to excess, eat a high-fat, high-sugar, low-nutrient diet etc. As discussed throughout this book, over time, unhealthy habits result in a degeneration of the human body. Detoxification is a part of the recipe for maintaining health, but it is not a reset button for the Cumulative Effect. You need all of the Habits of Health working in concert in order to get well soon and stay well!

In a Nutshell: The Detox Your Body Rules
1. Live on nature's harvest and drink plenty of clean water.
2. Break a sweat as often as possible.
3. Get into a routine that allows you to move your bowels at least two times per day.
4. Build into your routine some combination of skin exfoliation, deep breathing and antioxidant supplementation.
5. Do a two to three-day juice fast at least once per year.

A Word about the 8 Habits of Healthy People
If you are beginning to worry about the challenge of adopting these habits, don't. There is an activity in Part III of this book that will help you prioritize the habits that you need to adopt and a simple approach to

help you adopt them and make them a routine part of your life. In addition, there is an entire website (www.habitsofhealth.com) devoted to helping you adopt The 8 Habits of Healthy People with an abundance of great resources.

Chapter 12

Give it a Rest

What happens in the mind of man is always reflected in the disease of his body.

René Dubos

In his bestseller *Ordering Your Private World*, Gordon MacDonald asks his readers, "Has it occurred to you how often we talk about our fatigue? I sometimes have the feeling that if I don't tell my friends how tired I am they will doubt I am doing anything worthwhile... How did we get to a day when stress and fatigue are almost a badge of success?"

Very often, our busy lives are what create our bad habits in the first place. We live in a competitive, winner-take-all world and our lives reflect it. We strive for achievement and long for material possessions, so we study all the time or work too much. With little time to spare for life's "unproductive" tasks, we end up eating junk food on the go, skipping exercise, sleeping less, fueling up on caffeine and sugar and encountering more and more stress along the way. Before we know it, we have entrenched ourselves into a series of interconnected bad habits.

"It's okay," we tell ourselves. "I am working towards a goal and successful people are busy." Unfortunately, every day that you work towards your goal and follow those bad health habits, your health slips a little. Eventually, you wind up on your custom marble floor, grasping your chest in pain and regretting the choices that you've made.

Sound like one of those scary stories that your parents told you to get you to brush your teeth or not skip school? It's not. Look around you. Chronic diseases have reached epidemic proportions in the developed world and it is a direct result of the bad habits that get built around a busy, working lifestyle. Two of the hallmarks of the busy workaday life are lack of sleep and a load of stress.

If you are like me, you have a hard time prioritizing sleep. My mind is always going to my to-do lists and I have a very hard time truly shutting down. With three small children, a company to manage, books to write and a house full of remodeling projects, it is very tempting for me to steal time from sleep in order to get more done. People like me have a foolish pride about how busy they are because our society associates busy-ness with importance (I often wonder if that is how "business" got its name). So, not only are we busy, but we think rest is for the retired, under-employed or unsuccessful.

In addition, people like me tend to also underestimate the importance of stress management. Most people, men in particular, view stress as a natural part of the pressure of achievement. We have an I-eat-stress-for-breakfast mentality and just grind through it. Stress management is for the faint of heart and weak of character, we tell ourselves. Being able to carry stress and not crack is a badge of professional maturity in most circles.

The truth is, there are considerable health consequences with this type of living. Lack of sleep and persistent stress have a tangible negative impact on your health. Among other health consequence, both lack of sleep and persistent stress significantly suppress the immune system, increasing vulnerability to sickness and, in time, chronic disease.

Sleep
Getting even 30 minutes less sleep than your body needs per night can lead to the accumulation of a "sleep debt," which has both short and long-term consequences for mood, physical and mental performance and overall health. A sleep debt can make you more prone to accidents and impair your thinking and judgment and it can even be a causal factor for obesity. In addition, without adequate rest, you don't produce enough serotonin, which is believed to play an important role in the regulation of anger, aggression, body temperature, mood, sleep, sexuality, and appetite.

Most importantly though, sleep modulates immune function and a lack of sleep suppresses your immune system, reducing your body's ability to fight off sickness and disease. The idea that prolonged sleep deprivation alters immune function is probably not a shock to you. However, knowing that a *single* night of shortened or interrupted sleep suppresses the immune system might come as a surprise. In recent years, scientists have discovered a measurable reduction of natural and cellular immune response after a single night of accumulated sleep debt. Fortunately, the immune suppression is not permanent. Scientists also found that immune response recovers once a normal sleep pattern resumes.

Scientists can't say with certainty how sleep bolsters immune function, but they have shown that sleep repairs a suppressed immune system like nothing else can. No doubt this is why I have found that sleep is the fastest acting antibiotic. Over the years, I have found that my best defense against colds and flu is going to sleep as soon as I feel the symptoms coming on. As soon as I notice sore throat, fever, swollen glands, etc., I go home, crawl in bed and sleep for as long as I can.

The amount and quality of the sleep you get is a critical factor in your overall health, particularly your immune health and your ability to fight off The Cumulative Effect. The average person needs 7-8 hours a night, but it differs for every person. You would do well to get plenty of restful sleep every night and I recommend that you turn to sleep early and often in the event that you do feel an illness coming on. Below are some tips to help you get an adequate amount of restful sleep every night.

Go to bed. The most important thing about healthy sleep is routine: try to go to sleep and wake up at the same time every day – including weekends. As described earlier in this book, your body "wants" to be in a routine and when it is, it craves the stimulus provided by that routine. Since the beginning of human time, people have gone to bed with the setting of the sun and awakened with the rising of the sun. Our bodies' natural rhythms are adjusted to this schedule. If you go to sleep at the same time every night, your body will expect that and allow you to more easily fall into a deep, restful sleep. If you wake up at the same time every day, your body will expect that too, and you will rouse more alert, rested and energetic. When you break from your pattern, even just for the weekends, your body and brain do not get the stimulus they are expecting and you don't feel rested. Of course we will all have the occasional adjustments to our schedule, but try stick to your routine as much as possible. You will feel more rested for it.

In addition, try to establish a regular, relaxing bedtime routine such as taking a hot bath, reading or listening to calming music. I also recommend that you use your bedroom for sleep and sex only, keeping work, computers, etc. out of the bedroom. The bedroom should be a calming environment that is comfortable and conducive to sleep. You should also finish eating and complete all exercise at least two hours before your regular bedtime and avoid caffeine, alcohol and tobacco products late in the day.

...In a good bed. Make sure that your bed provides you optimal comfort and support. First, ensure that your bed is well suited for restful sleep (not too small, too squeaky, etc.). Next, I recommend that you buy the best mattress and box spring you can afford. Research shows that the quality of a mattress and box spring directly impact the quality of sleep. You will spend 1/3 of your life in bed, so it should be the one piece of furniture that you obsess over. Lastly, be sure to evaluate your mattress and box spring every five to seven years to ensure they still provide optimal comfort and support.

I also recommend that you discard uncomfortable bedding and pillows and invest in soft, comfortable bedding. I use and highly recommend down-filled bedding. Down bedding and pillows are amazingly comfortable and have an unusual ability to be cool to the touch and keep you warm at the same time. Finally, keep the room cool, quiet and dark. This will promote deep, restful sleep.

Stress
Life is full of challenges and obstacles, and sometimes the pressure is hard to manage. When we feel overwhelmed or unsure of how to meet the demands placed on us, we experience physical and emotional stress. In certain circumstances, stress can be a good thing. Stress can give you the motivation to push through a demanding situation or it can give you a burst of energy to overcome a challenging obstacle. However, when stress becomes commonplace in your life, it is a very real threat to your health.

The simplest definition of stress is that it is an emotional and physical response to events that we do not expect or want. It results from a disparity between what you experience (real or imagined) and what you expect. Stress can be brought on by stressors such as deadlines, relationship difficulties, conflict, births, deaths, marriage, pain, unemployment, a shortage of money and many other situations.

When something is different than we expect it to be, our brains launch a biological stress response in our bodies. This response is often called the fight or flight response. It causes the release of adrenaline and other hormones, a reaction that helped man survive the many threats to his wellbeing throughout history. In addition, it redirects blood to the brain and large muscles to improve mental acuity and strength; increases blood sugar to provide for energy; and increases the blood's clotting ability to reduce bleeding that could occur during said fighting or flight-ing. We feel this fight or flight response as an increased heart rate and blood pressure, dry mouth, sweating, enlarged pupils and sleeplessness.

The stress response is what helped our ancestors survive the many threats to their lives, improving their ability to fight or flee from danger. Today, however, most stressors are emotional, rather than physical. Losing a job or getting into a disagreement with a family member are stressful situations, but neither calls for physically fighting or fleeing. Unfortunately, our bodies can't make this distinction and they react as if we were surprised by a giant grizzly bear. We release the same hormones that enabled our ancestors to think quicker, see better, run faster, jump further, hit harder and hear more clearly than they could only seconds earlier. And while this response surely saved the lives of many of our ancestors, it is not necessary or helpful in most modern situations that create stress.

For the average person, emotions trigger the fight or flight stress response several times every day and, unfortunately, the stress response doesn't shut off once the stressor is removed. Instead, stress hormones, heart rate, blood pressure and blood sugar remain elevated. And, not surprisingly, repeated activation of the stress response takes a heavy toll on the body.

Persistent or repeated stress response (the biological response described above) can damage the cardiovascular system and suppress the immune system, reducing one's ability to fight the Cumulative Effect. Physical symptoms of stress include digestive problems, irregular heartbeat, shortness of breath, chest pain, high blood pressure, changes in sleep, headaches, weight gain or loss, teeth grinding or jaw clenching, overdoing leisure activities such as shopping, substance abuse, losing your temper and overreacting to unexpected problems. Mental symptoms of the body's biological stress response include repetitive or racing thoughts, desire to escape, poor judgment and decision making, loss of objectivity, hypersensitivity, anxiety, irritability, lack of confidence, apathy and even depression. Persistent and repeated stress response can contribute in a significant way to hypertension, strokes, heart attacks, diabetes, ulcers, cancer, obesity, autoimmune disorders and other chronic, degenerative conditions.

Stress is a real and tangible threat to your health. It is not some ethereal concept behind which weak people hide. It is a natural, physiological response that exists to preserve human life in emergencies. Unfortunately, the dynamic nature of our modern lifestyle differs greatly from the comparatively routine lifestyles of our ancient ancestors. As a result, that physiological response, which was intended for the rare emergency in a routine life, is now triggered frequently because very little in our lives is routine and many things differ from our expectations. The frequency with which the physiological stress response occurs today has genuine health consequences and no one is immune. Therefore, it is important to know how to deal with stress to minimize its impact on your health.

Dealing with Stress

Life comes with stress. Stress is an unavoidable consequence of life and you should not expect to live a stress-free life. Instead, you should strive to 1) prevent stressors from acting on you to cause a stress response, and 2) learn to effectively deal with the stressors that you cannot prevent from acting on you. Reinhold Niebuhr was a Protestant Christian theologian best known for relating religion to the reality of modern politics and diplomacy in the United States. His most well-known contribution may be the serenity prayer which is particularly applicable when discussing how to effectively deal with stress.

> "Grant me the courage to change the things I can change, the serenity to accept the things I can't change, and the wisdom to know the difference."

There are some stresses that you can prevent from acting on you by changing your habits – such as preparing for a deadline early – and others that you must simply learn to effectively manage, like the loss of a loved one. Knowing the difference is critical to successfully dealing with stress.

Prevent stressors from acting on you. Preventing stress involves identifying the sources of nagging stress in your life, determining whether or not the stressor can be eliminated, and finding ways to avoid them or reduce their impact. Most likely, the same handful of situations cause you stress repeatedly – being late, having more work than time, having more expenses than money, etc. For most people, the 80/20 rule applies to stress. If you can eliminate the top three stressors in your life, you can probably eliminate 70% - 80% of the stress responses in your life.

You may have more stressful situations to face than these nagging stressors, but the quantity of stress responses that you encounter is far more harmful than the severity of individual stress responses when you consider that the physiological response is similar in both. If you experience stress as a result of being late three times per week, you will experience the physiological stress response 156 times per year and likely more than 10,000 times in your life. Experiencing conflict with a coworker or boss might cause a more severe stress response because it is usually very unexpected and unpleasant, but it may only happen once or twice per year (any more and you should probably find a new job!)

Once you have honestly identified the sources of repeated stress, create a plan to change your habits or to remove yourself from those situations. Then, earnestly work that plan and assess the frequency with which you encounter that stressor. This will tell you how well your plan is working. As an example, below are some steps for a plan to eliminate the most common self-inflicted stressor – poor time management.

- Plan Ahead – Make a reasonable schedule for yourself and include down time in your schedule. Do not over-commit yourself on paper or to others. Becoming overwhelmed is the most common, stressful mistake. Instead, make a very short list (three or less) of the tasks you *have* to do, and then schedule time to complete them one-by-one. You can always do more if you find yourself with extra time.
- Be Realistic – All too often, we overestimate our ability to get things done and don't schedule enough time for each task. Be conservative and give yourself more than enough time to complete a task. Also, resist the temptation to schedule things back-to-back. This creates unnecessary pressure to finish a task by a certain time.
- Chunk Your Time – Aim to work in short, intensive periods and plan to rest in between. Break big assignments into smaller, more manageable tasks so that you don't feel overwhelmed and sit helplessly trying to figure out how to get started.
- Don't Procrastinate – Rank your tasks by priority and then schedule them that way, doing the most important tasks first. No matter how

unpleasant an important task is, don't put it off. Putting off important tasks always creates worry and anxiety the rest of the day as you anticipate having to do the task in less and less available time.

Effectively deal with stress that you cannot prevent from acting on you. Some of the stress in our lives cannot be eliminated. It must simply be managed as effectively as possible to reduce the negative health affects associated with the stress response. Unlike the stressors described above, this kind of stress does not typically show up in our lives consistently. Unpreventable stress is most often a surprise – like the loss of a loved one – but it can also hang around and become a nagging stressor, like the loss of a job that leads to financial woes.

In the case of stress that cannot be prevented, you must identify the physical symptoms that accompany it and learn stress reduction techniques to reduce its effects. Many stress relievers work because they counteract the physiological fight or flight response. Others work because of the placebo effect that comes from having faith in the procedure. Still others reduce stress because they reduce feelings of helplessness and provide a sense of control over the stressor. Below are some stress reduction recommendations and techniques:

- Have a Stress Relief Valve – Recognize the symptoms of stress and, when they happen, be diligent about taking immediate steps to relieve the stress in order to reduce the physiological stress response and lessen the negative health impact. When you feel stress coming on, try taking a short break to meditate, pray, take a walk, listen to music, play with a pet, do progressive muscular relaxation exercises or deep breathing exercises. If stress becomes severe and consistent, take a longer break and treat yourself to a massage, do yoga or tai chi, or enjoy one of your hobbies. No matter what the circumstances, don't treat stress with alcohol. Using alcohol to relieve stress can lead to dependency and other health problems.
- Use a Sounding Board – Having someone to share your thoughts and feelings with can help clear your mind and help you think through problems. Having a spouse, friend, coworker, family member or counselor that you can talk with openly and confidentially can help you see your problems differently and more objectively.
- Stick to an Exercise Routine – Exercise is proven to reduce stress and even protect against the negative health effects of stress. As recommended in an earlier chapter, you should find a way to be

active several times per week. During times of high stress, choose physical activity that is fun to you. Instead of climbing on the *stairmonster*, play a game of basketball with friends, climb the rock wall at the gym or ride your bike at the park.

- Get plenty of Sleep – As discussed earlier in this chapter, tiredness increases irritability and reduces your ability to reason. As a result, difficult situations cause more stress than they would when you are thinking rationally.

There is a great deal of irony in the notion that a physiological response designed to save our lives is now contributing to our demise. The world has changed faster than our bodies have been able to adapt and this physiological relic persists, creating a health risk that must be managed. In order to live a healthy life, stress has to be understood, identified and dealt with.

Giving it a Rest

Both persistent stress and lack of sleep suppress the immune system and contribute in a meaningful way to the epidemic of chronic illness that we are experiencing today. Our fast-paced, busy, upwardly mobile culture creates a lot of stress and causes us to think of rest as unproductive and sleep as inconvenient. Society views the type-A, hard-driving personality as a positive in the professional world and these people tend to be the ones who are rewarded with financial success. This reinforces the drive for productivity and undermines the notion that rest and stress management are necessary for good health. Building healthy sleep and stress management habits will noticeably improve your health and help to keep you well for a lifetime. If you are one of the many millions of people who steals time away from sleeping hours to invest in your productive life or if you have ignored the nagging stress in your life, make changing these habits a priority.

In a Nutshell: The Give it a Rest Rules

1. Have a daily routine. Sticking to a routine will improve the quality of your sleep and reduce the amount of stress in your life due to poor time management.
2. Get 7 to 8 hours of sleep every night.
3. Be active. People who exercise a few times a week sleep better and handle stress more effectively.

4. Identify the preventable stress in your life and create a plan to eliminate it. Preventing the three most common stressors in your life from acting on you will probably eliminate more than 70% of the stress you encounter.

PART III

Get Well Soon

.

In Part I of this book, you read about the epidemic of chronic illness and how your habits determine your participation in that epidemic. In Part II, you learned about the eight habits that determine human health. Now you will learn how to adopt those habits and make them a permanent part of your life. But before you can feel confident about making the effort to adopt these habits, you need to feel certain that these *are* the habits of healthy people.

I was once asked, "How can *you*, a person with no medical training, possibly know that there are eight little habits that can prevent such complex diseases?" Part of this question is a good question, and part of it is a bad question. The part about medical training, in my view, is wholly irrelevant. The many dedicated people with extensive medical training and medical school degrees haven't been able to prevent these complex diseases from ravaging our population. So, in my view, medical training is not a prerequisite for probing the causes of chronic disease. Asking how I could know which habits to choose *is a good question.*

Once you let go of (or, as in my case, give up on) the sick care, break-fix paradigm and get comfortable with the idea that there are a finite set of behaviors that need to be repeated regularly and consistently in order for humans to maintain their health, you naturally focus on what those finite behaviors are. I understood this idea and set out to identify the set of finite behaviors (habits) for my own benefit. Frankly, I wasn't targeting a number. The point isn't that there are eight behaviors (habits) … or seven … or nine. After almost losing my life to cancer, my health was my priority, and I would have done it if there were 16 or 23.

After a great deal of research, a significant effort to cross reference a long list of disparate recommendations, a lot of trial and error on myself, and even collapsing a few habits together, I came up with eight. But the question I was asked was, how do I know that these are *the* finite set of behaviors that need to be repeated regularly and consistently in order for humans to maintain their health. Couldn't swimming in ice cold spring water every day be a healthy habit? Couldn't hanging upside down for 20 minutes per day be a healthy habit?

They could be. The habits that I ultimately selected for this book, however, are the ones that were broadly supported in my research and proven to directly target the factors leading to the Cumulative Effect. I believe that the Eight Habits of Healthy People cover the vast majority of the behaviors that need to be repeated regularly and consistently in order for humans to maintain their health.

To prove to myself that I was not out in left field with this conclusion, I reviewed the prevention recommendations of the leading degenerative disease organizations – the American Cancer Society, The American Lung Association and The American Heart Association. Although I think they should do a great deal more in the area of prevention, they are the leading authorities on causation and disease. I am pleased to report that their recommendations generally support the conclusions that I have drawn with a few notable exclusions that commercially funded science is not ready to acknowledge. I have included a synopsis below:

On the American Cancer Society website, I reviewed the recommendations for preventing many of the most common types of cancer (breast, colorectal, lung, prostate, esophageal, stomach, etc.). The combined list of prevention recommendations are:

- Limit intake of animal products, especially red meat and high-fat dairy products.
- Eat 7 to 13 servings of vegetables and fruits each day.
- Avoid all forms of tobacco.
- Restrict alcohol consumption.
- Avoid obesity.
- Increase your physical activity.

On the American Lung Association website, I found the following prevention recommendations:

- Choose an overall balanced diet with foods from all major food groups, emphasizing a variety of fruits, vegetables and grains.
- Limit your intake of foods high in calories or low in nutrition including foods like soft drinks and candy that have a lot of sugars.
- Limit foods with a high content of saturated fat and cholesterol. Limit trans fatty acids.
- Limit alcohol consumption to no more than one drink per day for women and two drinks per day for men.
- Achieve a healthy body weight.
- Maintain a level of physical activity that achieves fitness and balances energy expenditure with caloric intake.
- Achieve a desirable cholesterol level.

- Achieve a desirable blood pressure level.

On the American Heart Association website, I found the following prevention recommendations:

- Eat a variety of nutritious foods from all the food groups.
- Eat less of the nutrient-poor foods.
- Use up at least as many calories as you take in.
- Don't smoke tobacco — and stay away from tobacco smoke.

With a few important exceptions, the prevention habits I recommend are aligned with the recommendations of the major disease associations. All this really proves, though, is that the habits that make you healthy do not require special training to discover. The key to health does not lie in the discovery of mysterious rituals practiced by ancient cultures in faraway lands. The key to health is in the *adoption of healthy habits.*

Chapter 13

Make a Plan

When health is absent, wisdom cannot reveal itself, art cannot manifest, strength cannot fight, wealth becomes useless, and intelligence cannot be applied.

Herophilus

Look around you. Take a look at the people in your life. It shouldn't take long for you to conclude, as I have, that we are sick as a species and getting worse.

The trouble is that it is hard to convince us of the truth. We want to believe we are healthier. We don't want to think that we are going backwards in any area, particularly not the health of our species. We want to believe in human ingenuity and man's dominion over the earth and everything in it. And we are marketed into believing that we are healthier because we regularly hear that human life expectancy is increasing and we are bombarded by propaganda from the drug companies and disease associations that leads us to believe that we are healthier.

It is just not true.

It took a long time for people to begin to admit that we were destroying the earth's environment and its atmosphere, but we eventually did because of overwhelming scientific evidence. The same data exists about the epidemic of disease overtaking our species. We simply need to review the evidence and the truth will emerge from the propaganda.

I have found that most people know this even if they don't acknowledge it with their actions. People walk around knowing that they are making poor health choices. It haunts them in their subconscious mind. The first thing people do when they see someone they haven't seen for 15 or 20 years after saying, "hello" is to make excuses about their weight.

I am encouraged that most people seem to know they are living unhealthy lives. I am encouraged because, as with any personal change program, the first step in the path to change is always the same. You must first acknowledge that you have a problem and admit that you have something to do with it. This step, the admission of a self-inflicted problem, is so important with the Habits of Health. Admitting this problem is critical if you intend to make a permanent change in your life.

If you *don't* believe this, *don't* go any further. If you don't really believe that your habits determine your health, and not some break-fix medical care system, you can't make this program stick. You will make a half-hearted effort and fail – and I don't want you telling people that this program doesn't work. So, if that's you, put this book down and go have a HoHo. Better yet, find the sickest person you know and trade them this book for their HoHo.

I'm dead serious.

If you *do* fess up to this – if you can see the poor health habits that have evolved in your life, if you can visualize the sickness at the end of the path that you are on, if you can think of sickness and disease as an enemy to be defeated – I applaud you. You are ready to make a Habits of Health plan and take the first step towards controlling your health.

For those of you who are ready to make changes in your habits, you need to start with a plan. Below, I have described the three steps for building your Habits of Health Plan (Prioritize, Assess and Select). Following the descriptions, there is an exercise for each step to help you put together your plan.

Since you create/change a few habits at a time, over time, this will be the first of several plans you make. I strongly recommend you do not skip the step of building a Habits of Health Plan each time because it is of critical importance.

Please note that if you need additional copies of the exercises below or cannot/would prefer not to write in this book, the exercises can be downloaded on our Website at www.habitsofhealth.com.

Prioritize – To be successful at changing your habits, you must be ready for change. If you have made it this far in the book, you are no doubt full of motivation to change your habits. Yet, if you are like most people, you are conflicted about where to start.

You are probably concerned about your health and you see many opportunities to improve your habits, but you need some help deciding where to start. Below, you will find a short questionnaire that will help you to narrow in on your goals and priorities.

Assess – In order to know what to fix, you have to know what is broken. However, knowing what is broken requires an objective assessment of your habits, which is difficult for most people. Although we generally know what our bad habits are, we often don't recognize or acknowledge how often we actually follow them.

For this reason, I created the Habits of Health Self-Assessment, a private, personal lifestyle diagnostic. This tool will help you objectively rate your habits.

It is tempting to skip the questionnaire and go right to the self-assessment, but resist that temptation. It is important to do these exercises in order. It is also important to remember to be honest in these exercises. You need an objective assessment of your habits and being honest is the only way to get one. Only you will see the results. If you are worried about someone else seeing your results after you read the book, tear the exercise pages out and put them somewhere private.

Select – Once you have prepared yourself mentally for adopting new habits and completed an objective assessment of your current habits, you are ready to identify the habits that you plan to change. The final exercise in this chapter builds off of the questionnaire and the Habits of Health Self-Assessment to help you select the habits that you plan to address first. Once you finish this exercise, you will have selected one to two habits that you plan to change.

If this is your first time through this process, I highly recommend that you start with one bad habit, apply my habit-change methodology to that habit, and then once that habit has become a healthy habit, move on to the next one. Changing habits takes focus and motivation. The more habits that you try to change at once, the more energy it takes and the lower your chances of success.

Rome wasn't built in a day. You can't change all of your habits in one shot. You will have to give yourself time to make these changes. If you try to change too much, too fast, you will continually fail, get discouraged and quit trying. Neither of us wants that. Instead, channel that motivation and energy to change into one or two habits at a time. If you do this, you will have a far greater chance of permanently adopting new healthy habits.

Prioritize Exercise: Health Questionnaire

You will need a pencil for this exercise.

List your top three reasons (motivations) for wanting to be healthier:

1. _____

_____

2. _____

_____

3. _____

_____

Examples:
- I want to protect my children from the pain of worrying about sick parents.
- I want to be an example of healthy living for my children and their children.

List your top three health goals:

1. _____

2. _____

3. _____

Examples:
- To avoid degenerative disease.
- To reduce my sick days at work and my healthcare costs.

List your top three health concerns:

1. _____

2. _____

3. _____
Examples:
- A chronic disease that reduces my lifespan or quality of life.
- Becoming a burden to my family.

List the two to three healthiest people you know and what you think makes them healthy:

_____

_____

_____

_____

Examples:
- Jim Smith – He is a runner, a vegetarian and is knowledgeable about nutrition.
- Allison Frost – She eats well and uses yoga and meditation to reduce her stress.

List the two to three *unhealthiest* people you know and what you think makes them *unhealthy*:

_____

_____

_____

_____

Examples:

- Reid Anderson – He drinks too much alcohol, eats too much fast food and has poor sleep habits.
- Carmen White – She is overweight and lives on snack food and diet soda.

Congratulations! You are finished with this exercise. Next, you will complete the Assess exercise.

You will need a pencil for this exercise.

What follows is a self assessment that is intended to help you assess the impact that your habits have on your health and to help you prioritize the habits you want to change. There are three important guidelines to remember while you are taking this self test:

- Consider your habits over the last year. Your answers to this self test should represent your <u>average over the last twelve months</u>. For example, if the question is about the number of times that you exercise per week, you should estimate the average number of times you have exercised per week over the last twelve months and pick the answer that most closely matches your estimate.

- Be honest. No one is going to see your answers. Answering these questions as accurately as you can gives you the best chance of understanding the impact that your habits have on your body.

- Don't be alarmed. If you have answered questions honestly and you don't like the way this self assessment is shaping up, keep going and be honest. There is a tendency to begin to go easier on yourself after you have given a few answers that you don't like. Don't do it. Being honest on this assessment is an important step towards getting healthy. In the next chapter, you will learn how to change those habits and improve your results.

1. How many servings of fruit do you consume on average (1 serving = 1 whole apple, peach, pear, banana, orange or grapefruit, 1 cup of berries, melon, pineapple, mixed fruit, apple sauce or 100% fruit juice, or ½ cup of dried fruit)?

    ( ) A. Four or more servings per day
    ( ) B. Two to three servings per day
    ( ) C. One serving per day
    ( ) D. Two to six servings per week
    ( ) E. Four or fewer servings per month

2. How many servings of vegetables, beans and peas do you consume on average (1 serving = 1 cup of raw, cooked, fresh, frozen, canned, dried, whole, cut-up or mashed vegetables, beans or peas or 100% vegetable juice)?

        ( ) A. Four or more servings per day
        ( ) B. Two to three servings per day
        ( ) C. One serving per day
        ( ) D. Two to six servings per week
        ( ) E. Four or fewer servings per month

3. How many different colors of fruits, vegetables, beans and peas do you consume (vegetables and fruits can be green, yellow, red, orange, blue, purple, white and brown)?

        ( ) A. Five or more colors per day
        ( ) B. Three to four colors per day, but the colors vary from day to day.
        ( ) C. Three to four colors per day, but the colors *don't* vary from day to day.
        ( ) D. One to two colors per day, but the colors vary from day to day.
        ( ) E. One to two colors per day, but the colors *don't* vary from day to day.

4. How many servings of whole grains, nuts and seeds do you consume on average (1 serving = one cup of whole grain cereal, oatmeal, brown rice, wild rice or whole grain crackers, nuts or seeds; one slice of whole grain bread or cornbread; one whole grain muffin, bagel, pancake, tortilla or English muffin; or three cups of popcorn)?

        ( ) A. Four or more servings per day
        ( ) B. Two to three servings per day
        ( ) C. One serving per day
        ( ) D. Two to six servings per week
        ( ) E. Four or fewer servings per month

5. What % of your edible groceries by food volume would you estimate are certified organic or wild caught on average (consider all dairy, meat, poultry, eggs, fish, seafood, fruit, vegetables, soy products, bread, cereal, nuts, sauces and spreads, juice, wine, beer, coffee, tea, condiments, spices and ingredients like sugar, flour and cooking oil)?

      ( ) A. >50%
      ( ) B. 34% - 50%
      ( ) C. 21% - 33%
      ( ) D. 10% to 20%
      ( ) E. Less than 10%

6. How many ounces of filtered water or spring water do you estimate that you consistently consume on a daily basis (water that has been filtered by a modern water filter or water originating from a natural spring)?

      ( ) A. Male: >96 ounces, Female: >64 ounces
      ( ) B. Male: 89-96 ounces, Female: 57-64 ounces
      ( ) C. Male: 73-88 ounces, Female: 41-56 ounces
      ( ) D. Male: 64-72 ounces, Female: 32-40 ounces
      ( ) E. Male: <64 ounces, Female: <32 ounces

7. How often do you eat foods that contain added sugar, high-fructose corn syrup or artificial sweetener? (1 serving = 1 cup of breakfast cereal, 1 pastry, muffin, breakfast bar or doughnut; 1 small candy bar, 1 small handful of cookies, candy or sweet snacks; 1 brownie, 1 small slice of cake or pie, 1 small scoop of ice cream, etc.):

      ( ) A. Three or more servings per day
      ( ) B. Two servings per day
      ( ) C. One serving per day
      ( ) D. Two to six servings per week
      ( ) E. Four or fewer servings per month

8. How often do you eat packaged snack food (1 serving = 1 cup of most anything from a snack machine, convenience store, most store-bought salty or sugary snacks)?

      ( ) A. Three or more servings per day
      ( ) B. Two servings per day
      ( ) C. One serving per day
      ( ) D. Two to six servings per week
      ( ) E. Four or fewer servings per month

9. How often do you eat a meal containing fried foods or a high-fat meat like bacon, hot dogs, sausage, steak or ground beef?

    ( ) A. Two or more times per day

    ( ) B. Once per day

    ( ) C. Two to six times per week

    ( ) D. Two to four times per month

    ( ) E. Once per month or less

10. How often do you eat prepared food from a convenience store or from a fast food/quick service restaurant (McDonalds, Burger King, Wendy's Dairy Queen, Pizza Hut, Domino's, Dunkin Donuts, KFC, Taco Bell, Quizno's, Little Caesars, Long John Silvers, etc.)?

    ( ) A. Two or more times per day

    ( ) B. Once per day

    ( ) C. Two to six times per week

    ( ) D. Two to four times per month

    ( ) E. Once per month or less

11. How often do you eat food from a table service or buffet-style restaurant (eat in or take out)?

    ( ) A. Three meals per day

    ( ) B. Two meals per day

    ( ) C. One meal per day

    ( ) D. Two to six meals per week

    ( ) E. Four or fewer meals per month

12. How often do you consume unfiltered municipal water-based drinks (1 serving of unfiltered municipal water based drink = 12 ounces of unfiltered tap water, home- or office-brewed coffee made with unfiltered water, convenience store and restaurant coffee or fountain soda, most canned or packaged soft drinks and juices, etc.)?

    ( ) A. Three or more servings per day

    ( ) B. Two servings per day

    ( ) C. One serving per day

    ( ) D. Two to six servings per week

    ( ) E. Four or fewer servings per month

13. How often do you drink beverages that contain added sugar, high-fructose corn syrup or artificial sweetener (1 serving = 12 ounces of soda, sweetened tea or coffee, flavored milk, most juices, sports drinks and energy drinks and many flavored waters)?

      ( ) A. Three or more servings per day
      ( ) B. Two servings per day
      ( ) C. One serving per day
      ( ) D. Two to six servings per week
      ( ) E. Four or fewer servings per month

14. How often do you consume caffeine (1 serving = 12 ounces of caffeinated coffee, tea, soda, or energy drink; 1 caffeine-containing energy pill, powder or supplement)?

      ( ) A. Five or more servings per day
      ( ) B. Three to four servings per day
      ( ) C. One to two servings per day
      ( ) D. Two to six servings per week
      ( ) E. Four or fewer servings per month

15. How often do you drink alcohol on average (1 serving = 12 ounces of beer or wine cooler, 8 ounces of wine, 1.5 ounces of liquor/ distilled spirits)?

      ( ) A. Three or more servings per day
      ( ) B. Two servings per day
      ( ) C. One serving per day
      ( ) D. Two to six servings per week
      ( ) E. Four or fewer servings per month

16. How often do you use tobacco products (1 time = 1 cigarette, 1 cigar, 1 pipe-full of tobacco or 1 pinch of smokeless tobacco)?

      ( ) A. Two or more times per day
      ( ) B. Once per day
      ( ) C. Two to six times per week
      ( ) D. Four or fewer times per month
      ( ) E. Never

17. How often do you use non-prescribed narcotics or controlled substances (marijuana, methamphetamine, ecstasy, cocaine, codeine, hydrocodone, oxycodone, heroin, etc.)?
     ( ) A. More than twice per month
     ( ) B. One to two times per month
     ( ) C. Four to eleven times per year
     ( ) D. One to three times per year
     ( ) E. Never

18. How many prescription drugs with at least one known side effect do you take (count each dose of each drug individually)?
     ( ) A. Two or more doses per day
     ( ) B. One dose per day
     ( ) C. Two to six doses per week
     ( ) D. Two to four doses per month
     ( ) E. One dose per month or less

19. How many over-the-counter drugs with at least one known side effect do you take (pain relievers like aspirin, ibuprofen and acetaminophen, cold medicine, sinus medicine, allergy medicine, etc. – count each dose of each drug individually)?
     ( ) A. Three or more doses per day
     ( ) B. Two doses per day
     ( ) C. One dose per day
     ( ) D. Two to six doses per week
     ( ) E. Four or fewer doses per month

20. How many traditional (non-organic) skin, hair, and beauty products do you use per day on average (consider shampoo, soap, cologne, perfume, deodorant, toothpaste, mouthwash, mousse, hair gel, hair spray, mascara, lipstick, blush, lotion, etc.)?
     ( ) A. Six or more products per day
     ( ) B. Five products per day
     ( ) C. Three to four products per day
     ( ) D. One to two products per day
     ( ) E. None

21. How many traditional (non-organic) household and commercial chemical products would you estimate that you use or come into long-term physical contact with during an average day (consider all household and commercial cleaners, detergents, soaps, polishes, waxes, paints, stains, inks, dyes, solvents, oils, fuels, caulks, sealants, pesticides, fertilizers, etc.)?

     ( ) A. Six or more products per day
     ( ) B. Five products per day
     ( ) C. Three to four products per day
     ( ) D. One to two products per day
     ( ) E. None

22. How often do you get angry or experience high stress on average (to a level that it takes more than ten minutes to settle down emotionally and get past the experience)?

     ( ) A. Three or more times per day
     ( ) B. Two times per day
     ( ) C. One time per day
     ( ) D. Two to six times per week
     ( ) E. Four or fewer times per month

23. What is your blood pressure on average? (Electronic blood pressure monitors are available at most grocery and drug stores. When measured with a blood pressure monitor, the first number shown, the systolic pressure, is the pressure generated when the heart contracts. The second number shown, the diastolic pressure, is the blood pressure when the heart is relaxed.)

     ( ) A. >180 (systolic) over >110 (diastolic)
     ( ) B. 160 to 180 (systolic) over 100 to 110 (diastolic)
     ( ) C. 140 to 160 (systolic) over 90 to 100 (diastolic)
     ( ) D. 130 to140 (systolic) over 85 to 90 (diastolic)
     ( ) E. 90 to 130 (systolic) over 60 to 85 (diastolic)

24. How many hours of deep, uninterrupted sleep do you estimate that you consistently get on a daily basis?

     ( ) A. > 8 hours
     ( ) B. 7.5 – 8 hours
     ( ) C. 7 – 7.5 hours
     ( ) D. 6.5 – 7 hours
     ( ) E. < 6.5 hours

25. How often do you have a bowel movement on average?
  ( ) A. Three or more times per day
  ( ) B. Two times per day
  ( ) C. One time per day
  ( ) D. Five to six times per week
  ( ) E. Four or fewer times per week

26. How often do you exfoliate (scrub) your entire body on average?
  ( ) A. Three times per week
  ( ) B. Two times per week
  ( ) C. One time per week
  ( ) D. One to three times per month
  ( ) E. Rarely or never

27. How often do you perspire to the point of moistening your clothing?
  ( ) A. Five or more times per week
  ( ) B. Four times per week
  ( ) C. Three times per week
  ( ) D. Two times per week
  ( ) E. Four or fewer times per month

28. How often do you exercise for 20 minutes or more (Exercise = brisk walking, jogging, cycling, swimming, tennis, soccer, weight lifting, stair trainer, elliptical trainer, etc. To be considered exercise for this question, it must substantially elevate the heart rate and sustain it. Activities such as golf and casual walking should not be counted for this question).
  ( ) A. Five or more times per week
  ( ) B. Four times per week
  ( ) C. Three times per week
  ( ) D. Two times per week
  ( ) E. Four or fewer times per month

29. Outside of exercise, how often are you physically active for 30 minutes or more (walking, lifting, carrying, gardening, house work, etc.)?
  ( ) A. Five or more times per week
  ( ) B. Four times per week
  ( ) C. Three times per week
  ( ) D. Two times per week
  ( ) E. Four or fewer times per month

30. What is your body mass index BMI (BMI = Your weight in pounds ÷ Your height in inches ÷ Your height in inches x 703 —or— BMI = Weight in kilograms ÷ Height in meters ÷ Height in meters)?
        ( ) A. > 32
        ( ) B. 30 – 32 or < 18.5
        ( ) C. 28 – 29
        ( ) D. 26 – 27
        ( ) E. 18.5 – 25

31. What is your waist-to-hip ratio (WHR) (This is calculated by dividing the smallest circumference of your natural waist [usually just above the belly button] by the circumference of your hips at the widest part of your buttocks)?
        ( ) A. >0.8 for a woman, >0.95 for a man
        ( ) B. 0.78 – 0.8 for a woman, 0.94 – 0.95 for a man
        ( ) C. 0.75 – 0.77 for a woman, 0.92 – 0.93 for a man
        ( ) D. 0.72 – 0.74 for a woman, 0.90 – 0.91 for a man
        ( ) E. <0.72 or less for a woman, <0.90 for a man

32. How many times did you get a cold or the flu in the last twelve months?
( ) A. Five or more times
( ) B. Four times
( ) C. Two to three times
( ) D. One time
( ) E. Never

Great work! Now that you have completed the Habits of Health Self Test, below is the key to use to grade yourself. Using the grading scale below, go back through the self test question by question and add up your score (start from zero). Note that it is helpful to write down your total score every five questions or so in case you lose track. You will be both adding and subtracting points as you go along and it is easy to lose count. Also note that you may end up with a positive or a negative total score at the end.

For questions 1 – 6 and 25 – 29, if you answered:
A. Add 4 points to your score.
B. Add 3 points to your score.
C. Add 2 points to your score.
D. Add1 point to your score.
E. Add 0 points to your score.

For question 24, if you answered
A. Add 4 points to your score.
B. Add 3 points to your score.
C. Add 0 points to your score.
D. Subtract 2 points from your score.
E. Subtract 4 points from your score.

For questions 7 – 23 and 30 – 32, if you answered:
A. Subtract 4 points from your score.
B. Subtract 3 points from your score.
C. Subtract 2 points from your score.
D. Subtract 1 point from your score.
E. Subtract 0 points from your score.

Once you have finished grading yourself, write down today's date and
your score in one of the fill in the blank areas provided below. There are
multiple lines provided so that you can take the Habits of Health self test
again and again to see how your habits are improving.

Date: _____   Score: _____

Date: _____   Score: _____

Date: _____   Score: _____

Now, using the Habits Rating Chart pictured below, identify where your
score puts you on the scale and read below the chart to learn more about
your rating. Please note that this is not intended to be an exact measure.
It is merely a directional measure of your habits.

Dangerous Habits	Unhealthy Habits	Neutral Habits	Healthy Habits	Elite Habits

-80 -72 -64 -56 -48 -40 -32 -24 -16 -8   0   8   16   24   32   40   48

Elite Habits: If your score is between 32 and 48, take a bow. You have elite habits and we can all learn from your example. Assuming you are not killed by a falling piano, you will likely live a long life that is free of chronic, degenerative disease. I hope you have ample retirement savings because you will probably need it!

Healthy Habits: If your score is between 8 and 32, congratulations. You have worked at being healthy and you are undoubtedly feeling the benefits. You, too, can expect a long, healthy life if you keep it up. There are a few areas where you can improve, but you knew what those were before you took this quiz.

Neutral Habits: If your score is between -8 and +8, your habits are basically neutral. Your habits are neither the source of your health nor the source of your sickness. You probably spend some time thinking about your health, but you have not made a concerted effort to change it. Although your habits are not the source of your sickness, the world in which you live adds to the Cumulative Effect in your body every day and without healthier habits, your defenses against sickness and disease will weaken over time.

Unhealthy Habits: If your score is between -48 and -8, you are living a life of unhealthy habits that is constantly chipping away at your overall health. This is probably not a surprise to you as the little voice in your head has been telling you all along that you needed to change your lifestyle. In fact, you are probably reading this book because you knew that your habits were a problem for you and you needed some help. Keep reading – help is on the way.

Dangerous Habits: If your score is between -80 and -48, check your pulse and your life insurance. Let's be honest, you live an indulgent, self-destructive lifestyle and you know it. You would not be surprised at all to learn that you have heart disease, diabetes or cancer. In fact, deep down, you expect to get that news at some point. You *have* to change your lifestyle if you want to even have a lifestyle. This book can help you, but you have to commit yourself to becoming healthy, which is something you have probably struggled with for a long time.

Congratulations. You are finished with this exercise. Next, you will complete the Select exercise.

Select Exercise: Identifying Habits

You will need a pencil for this exercise.

In this exercise, there are several steps. Read the instructions and follow each step in order. At the conclusion of this exercise, you will select the habits that you will work to change.

Step 1 – Go back through the Habits of Health Self-Assessment that you just completed and circle the question numbers of the five questions where you scored poorly that you *most* want to improve. If this is your first time through, I recommend that you prioritize the questions in which you are most disappointed with your answer (where you know you can do better). If you have been through this process at least once, I recommend that you prioritize the questions that you believe are most detrimental to your overall health.

Step 2 – To use this chart, follow the instructions on the next page.

	Reducing the Accumulated Toxins Already in Your Body	Preventing Toxins From Entering Your Body	Restoring Your Immune System	Promoting Healthy Cell & Tissue Regeneration
Live on Nature's Harvest Q: 1-4, 9-11	+	+		++
Drink From the Fountain of Health Q: 6, 12, 13	+	+		+
Be In-Dependent Q: 7, 8, 14, 15, 16-19		+	+	
Use Your Body Q: 28, 29	+			+
Carry the Right Weight Q: 30, 31	+		+	+
Live an Organic Lifestyle Q:5, 20, 21		++		++
Detoxify Your Body Q: 25-27	++		+	++
Rest and Relax Q: 22-24			++	+

All of the questions in the self-assessment correlate to one of the 8 Habits of Healthy People described in this book. The habits and the questions that correlate to them are listed in the chart on the previous page. Draw a star next to each habit in the chart that correlates to a question that you prioritized in Step 1 above.

As you will recall, the Cumulative Effect is driven by accumulated toxins in the body, a weakened immune system and reduced functioning of the body's life sustaining systems (illustrated in the picture below).

The Cumulative Effect

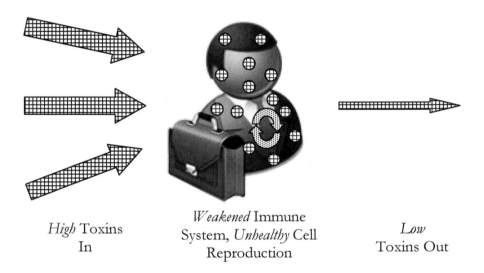

High Toxins
In

Weakened Immune
System, *Unhealthy* Cell
Reproduction

Low
Toxins Out

Each of the 8 Habits of Healthy People fight the Cumulative Effect by doing one or more of the following:
- Reducing the accumulated toxins already in your body
- Preventing toxins from entering your body
- Restoring your immune system so that it can fight for you
- Promoting healthy cell and tissue regeneration

For each of the habits that you starred in the chart, follow the rows out to the right to see the benefits that each habit has on fighting the factors that cause the Cumulative Effect in your body. One plus ("+") indicates that the habit causes some improvement. Two plusses ("++") indicates that the habit causes significant improvement.

Step 3 – Now it is time to choose one to two habits that you want to change. If your current Actual Score on the Habits of Health Self-Assessment (the score that you wrote down in the blank following the words "Actual Score" above) was between -80 and +8, I suggest that you select one to two habits to adopt that will give you some improvement across at least three of the factors driving the Cumulative Effect. If your current Actual Score was between +8 and +48, I suggest that you focus on improving the one to two habits where you need the most improvement (your least adopted/least routine habits).

Once you have chosen a habit or habits to adopt or improve, write it/them down in the blanks provided below. I strongly suggest that you not try to adopt/improve more than two at a time.

The Habit(s) of Health that I have chosen to adopt/improve are:

_____

_____

_____

_____

Congratulations. You have completed a Habits of Health Plan. This is an important preparatory step to changing your habits and changing your health.

Adopting the Eight Habits of Healthy people is a continuous improvement process. I encourage you to build a Habits of Health Plan each and every time that you take on a new set of habits. Take it from a guy that tried to change his habits with force of will alone: getting mentally prepared to take on change makes the change itself a lot easier.

For additional exercises to prepare you for adopting new habits, visit www.habitsofhealth.com. The exercises above, as well as several additional exercises not included in this book can be downloaded free of charge.

Chapter 14

Change U

We are what we repeatedly do. Excellence then, is not an act, but a habit.
Aristotle

It is time for another reality check.

If you are expecting me to tell you now that you can repeat a magic phrase four times and your habits will change, think again. Those commercials that promised that you could buy a piece of equipment, exercise for seven minutes per week and have a body like a swimsuit model – those were written by a dude who looks like Tom Arnold. The stud in the commercials works out at least two hours per day.

Changing your habits is not as easy as falling out of bed. It takes some commitment and work from you. My system is simple and it works, but it doesn't _do the work_. You do.

So, if you are not truly motivated to change your habits, then punt. I'm still serious. I don't want you to fail and tell people the program doesn't work.

But if you are motivated to change your habits, then do this thing. Your health is worth it.

In the last chapter, I outlined the three steps for building a Habits of Health Plan (Prioritize, Assess and Select) and provided exercises to help you through each step. In this chapter, I describe the two steps for executing your plan (Declare and Implement) and provide an exercise and a template to help you with these steps.

Declare – Now that you have identified the habits that you want to change, you need to get into the specifics of those habits. What are you going to change about that habit? How will your day be different? At what times? Where will you be at those times? What cues will remind you to implement those changes? What challenges will you face and how will you overcome them?

Former GE CEO Jack Welch is known for putting his managers on the spot for providing detailed answers to the question, "How do you intend to meet your goals?" Vowing to drink more clean water is not enough. Being specific means, for example, planning to drink sixteen ounces of filtered water during your morning workout; planning to fill your water jug as soon as you arrive at the office so you can drink twelve ounces before lunch, twelve ounces after lunch and eight ounces during your commute home from work; and then planning to drink another eight-ounce glass of water at bedtime. Being specific about what you intend to do forces you to think through the new behavior that you will follow in detail.

As you declare the specifics of your goals, use caution about being too ambitious. Radical changes in behavior are not easy to implement all at once. Set goals that you can really picture yourself achieving. For instance, don't set a goal of exercising two hours per day, six days per week if you are completely sedentary now. Instead, consider starting with twenty minutes per day, three days per week until that becomes a habit. On the next habit adoption round, you can increase the duration and frequency. Once you have achieved a few of your goals and your confidence increases, you can begin to stretch yourself a little bit.

In addition, remember that it is easier to modify an existing habit than to form a completely new one (this is what I call habit momentum). For example, it is easier to switch from drinking coffee to drinking green tea than it is to stop drinking coffee. It is easier to have a sweet piece of fruit when your body craves something sweet than it is to have nothing at all. As discussed, a habit is a routine that the body becomes accustomed to and expects. So, you can take advantage of the body's signals to perform the old routine, making the modification of old habits easier than forming completely new habits from scratch.

Lastly, it is important to know that certain habits, bad ones and good ones, form a framework that supports one another. The habit of over reacting to stress can support a habit of routinely drinking alcohol to "calm your nerves." Similarly, the habit of going to bed early lends itself to a morning exercise habit. As you declare the specifics of your plan, be on the lookout for existing habits that you can modify and good habits that support one another. It will make things easier for you.

To help you declare the specifics of your plan, there is a short questionnaire included below following the description of the Implement step. I recommend that you fill out this simple questionnaire for each habit that you intend to adopt.

Implement – If the following paragraphs seem familiar to you, it is because they are mostly reprinted from an earlier chapter. The concepts covered in these paragraphs are the cornerstone of this program, but they can be counter-intuitive, so I decided to simply include them again here.

As discussed earlier, the brain and body become accustomed, even dependent, upon the routines that you follow. When you try to change, the brain and body, expecting the stimulus provided by the customary routines, literally crave the expected stimulus. You sense the cravings – a candy bar after lunch, a cigarette during the commute, an evening on the couch instead of in the gym – and you probably fight them for a while. However, we all have moments of weakness, and we give in to the cravings. One moment of weakness justifies another and another, and pretty soon, you brain and body have pulled you back into the old routine.

Making sudden changes in lifestyle is difficult because of the principle of inertia. Things in motion tend to stay in motion. Our impatient, instant-gratification way of life leads us to think that sudden change is necessary, and our pride and stubbornness leads us to believe that it is possible. Adopting new habits or breaking old ones is nearly *im*possible to do using the cold turkey approach.

However, in our work, we found that things in motion can change direction little by little. The key to changing habits, it turns out, is subtleness, not suddenness. To change one's habits, one needs to be clever, not bold. The body must be re-trained to expect a new habit and this isn't achieved with resolve and force of will alone.

Breaking and forming habits is not hard, as we've come to believe. It is actually quite simple. It just requires a smarter approach: PRRT

- Progression – New habits are not formed all at once. Habit change is about subtleness, not suddenness. A ship at sail changes course slowly. Behavior change happens in much the same way.

- Routines – In order to adopt a habit, a person must have a structure in place that reminds him to follow certain behaviors. Without that structure, even with the best intentions, we tend to give in to our brain/body cravings for the stimulus it expects or to follow the path of least resistance. The most reliable support structure for permanently changing lifestyle habits is the daily routine.

- Repetition – Repetition is important in changing habits. The brain and body need to regularly practice the new habit in order for it to become an expected stimulus. Frequency makes a path a trail.

- Time – I bet you have heard the old adage, '21 days to make a habit.' It turns out that the time that it takes to make a habit depends upon several environmental factors that differ by person and habit. Generally, in 20 to 30 days, a consistently repeated behavior becomes habitual because your mind and body adjusts to it. It becomes the path of least resistance.

New Habit = Progression + Routines + Repetition + Time

The problem most people have when they try change their habits is that they try to do it all at once. They rely on willpower to try and overcome a routine and don't realize that they have to also overcome mental and physical cravings for their old habits. In order to be successful at changing your habits, you must progressively develop a new habit by leveraging an existing one that already has momentum (that your body is expecting). In addition, a routine that supports the new habit has to be formed so that old routines that helped to form the old habit don't pull you back. And, most importantly, you must repeat the changed habit for long enough that your body begins to expect the new stimulus. Most people don't have all of those elements when they set out to change their actions and, as a result, they often fail. PRRT takes advantage of the inertia of your existing habits and uses subtle changes, daily routines and repetition to change habits over time.

Included below (after the declaration exercise) is a PRRT Template. This is the tool you will use to guide you as you change your habits. . If you need additional copies of these exercises or cannot/would prefer not to write in this book, the exercises can be downloaded free of charge from www.habitsofhealth.com.

Declare Exercise: Habit Questionnaire

This exercise is intended to help you detail the specifics of a single habit that you plan to change. You will need a pencil for this exercise.

Habit:_____

     Example – Build my diet around nature's harvest.

Why do you want to start/end this habit?

_____

_____

_____

What does this habit consist of/entail?

_____

_____

_____

What specific behaviors/patterns/routines do you intend to follow in forming and keeping this habit?

_____

_____

_____

In what ways will this habit impact/change your day?

_____

_____

_____

At what times and where will you be when you expect to follow this habit?

_____

_____

_____

How will you consistently reinforce the adoption of this habit?

_____

_____

_____

What challenges do you expect to face in forming this habit?

_____

_____

_____

How do you plan to overcome those challenges?

_____

_____

_____

How will you hold yourself accountable to this habit building program?

_____

_____

_____

Who else will hold you accountable, helping you with this habit?

_____

_____

_____

Who is your role model for this habit and why?

_____

_____

_____

How will your measure your success in adopting this habit?

_____

_____

_____

When/how will you know that you have permanently adopted this habit?

_____

_____

_____

In what ways do you expect your health to improve as a result of this habit?

_____

_____

_____

What specific things will you do to make sure that you don't lose this habit once you complete the habit-building program?

_____

_____

_____

In the event that you do drop this habit, what will you do to re-adopt it?

_____

_____

_____

Congratulations. You are finished with this exercise. Next, you will move to the Implement step by creating a PRRT Template.

Implement Exercise: PRRT Template

You will need a pencil for this exercise.

This PRRT Template is intended for the adoption of a single habit. If you are adopting more than one habit (and I strongly recommend that you limit yourself to one at a time), use multiple PRRT Templates. Don't be intimidated by this template. It helps you lay things out in detail in order to make habit adoption much easier than you are accustomed to it being.

Habit:_____

     Example – Build my diet around nature's harvest.

Progression: Remember, effectively adopting habits is about subtleness, not suddenness. Big changes in lifestyle, adopted all at once, rarely stick.

Write down the three subtle behavior changes you will make in your life as you adopt this habit. The changes will be cumulative. In other words, you will add the first behavior change and later layer the second change on top of that and then include the third change.

For ideas on subtle behavior changes, go back to the chapter on the Habit of Health you are targeting in Part II of this book.

Most importantly, don't be too ambitious in the changes below. It will be demoralizing if you can't accomplish the changes you set out to.

Change 1:   _____

     Example - Stop eating packaged snack food and fried food.

Change 2:   _____

     Example - Begin eating fruit and whole grain cereal for breakfast.

Change 3:   _____

     Example - Begin building lunch around vegetables and whole grains.

Routine(s): You will not start adopting the behavior changes you identified above until week two. In week one of your PRRT program, you will simply observe your daily schedule. I suggest dividing a piece of paper into sevenths to keep track of your schedule for a week. Your goal is to identify existing routines in your daily life that you can use to reinforce the three behavior changes you listed above. Look for routines that will serve as an infrastructure to support a desired change.

Routine(s) to Support Change 1:

_____

_____

Example - During my morning coffee/quiet time, write down my menu for the day on a 4"x5" note card and pack healthy snacks into my brief case.

Routine to Support Change 2:

_____

_____

Example - Shop with healthy grocery list every Saturday morning before kids' sports activities, wash and cut up all fruit before family dinner on Saturday night so it can be served as desert at dinner and the extra is ready to eat for breakfast during the week ahead.

Routine to Support Change 3:

_____

_____

Example - Prepare vegetable-centered dinners two nights per week and eat leftovers for lunch; identify vegetable-centered dishes at frequented restaurants; buy frozen vegetable entrees to take to work when necessary.

Repetition and **T**ime: The PRRT approach to habit adoption sets aside seven weeks for adopting a habit or habits. If you look at the PRRT Table below, you will notice that there is a preparation phase, a buildup phase and an adoption phase. Week 1, the preparation phase, is for observing your daily schedule in search of supporting routines.

Weeks 2, 3 and 4, the buildup phase, is for adding the subtle changes you have identified. And weeks 5, 6 and 7, the adoption phase, provide 21 days for you to repeat the cumulative changes that you made in your behavior so that you can form a habit.

Using the PRRT Table is simple. Each cell in the table represents a day of the PRRT program. An empty cell is a day in which you are suppose to repeat a behavior or behaviors. A shaded cell is a day that you are not. For each empty cell, make a check mark when you repeat the desired behavior or behaviors. Your goal is to get six checks per week.

Remember: change 1, change 2 and change 3 are cumulative. They are not done instead of one another. So, you will only make a check mark if you successfully execute the cumulative behavior changes one or more times on the scheduled day. So, for example, in week 4, you will make a check if you accomplish changes 1, 2 and 3 on a given day of the week.

Also, since you only need six checks per week, I recommend that you schedule an off day. It has been my experience that everyone needs an off day or a "cheat" day to look forward to. When I am changing a habit, I make Friday my cheat day. Weekends may be harder for you to stay in a routine, so you might pick Saturday or Sunday. Pick a cheat day and mark it on the PRRT Table. Remember though, if you skip a day earlier in the week, that day becomes your cheat day for that week.

PRRT Table

	Preparation	Buildup			Adoption		
	Week 1	Week 2	Week 3	Week 4	Week 5-7		
	Observe	Change 1	Change 2	Change 3	Hold		
					5	6	7
Mon							
Tue							
Wed							
Thu							
Fri							
Sat							
Sun							

Example of a completed PRRT Table

	Preparation	Buildup			Adoption		
	Week 1	Week 2	Week 3	Week 4	Week 5-7		
	Observe	Change 1	Change 2	Change 3	Hold		
					5	6	7
Mon		☑	☑		☑	☑	☑
Tue		☑	☑	☑	☑	☑	☑
Wed		☑	☑	☑	☑	☑	☑
Thu			☑	☑		☑	☑
Fri		☑			☑		
Sat		☑	☑	☑	☑	☑	☑
Sun		☑	☑	☑	☑	☑	☑

PRRT is a simple, proven approach for adopting new habits. It takes advantage of the inertia of your existing habits and uses subtle changes, daily routines and repetition to change habits over time. PRRT makes forming new habits very predictable.

If you are like me, you may not think that you really need a system to change your habits. You may think you can do it on your own using your willpower alone, but don't let your ego get the best of you. If it were as simple as making a decision, you would have already changed your habits and you wouldn't be reading this book.

Embrace PRRT and start the process of building Habits of Health. The program was carefully designed based on years of experience in changing adult behavior. Follow each step as outlined above and you will have more success changing your habits than ever before.

Most of all, remember that you will never be perfect in your habits. You will have days when you do well and days when you do not do well. That's okay. As long as you have formed a lifestyle of interconnecting Habits of Health, the little slip ups and the planned cheating only make up about 5% - 10% of your overall activities. The other 90% - 95% of your activities will still be health-promoting and, as a result, you will experience a significant improvement in your overall health.

Is it better to do this program with someone else?

It depends on you, really. Some people are able to hold themselves accountable. Others have a higher chance of success in changing their habits if they have someone or some group hold them accountable to their commitments. If you do partner with one or more people, just be careful to choose people who have the same level of dedication that you do. If you choose to change your habits alone, I recommend that you tell someone close to you what you are doing so you have at least some accountability.

Why is cheating allowed?

Abstinence is difficult, especially when you are surrounded by the unhealthy habits that you have worked so hard to give up. That is why controlled cheating is encouraged. Remember, health is destroyed by the Cumulative Effect, which is the accumulation of the consequences of unhealthy habits and poor health choices – not a single chocolate covered cherry or a malt scotch on your annual golf trip.

Though cheating *can* very easily become a slippery slope, I still feel that the benefits of occasional controlled cheating outweigh the risks of slipping (slipping is the unconscious loss of momentum of a Habit of Health). To prevent cheating from turning into slipping, cheating must be controlled. It must have three parameters:

1. Cheating must be planned. Spontaneity is not necessarily a good thing when it comes to habits. Plan your cheating and resist it at all other times. It is far too easy to mentally justify an unplanned drink with your co-workers or a slice of birthday cake at a party. Soon all of those special occasions will have undone the healthy habits that you worked so hard to create. Plan ahead for regular cheating at specific times and in limited quantities.

2. Cheating must be isolated in time. Pick a time that you can regularly cheat. I allow myself to have a "junk" meal on Fridays. For me, this usually means Bar-B-Q. However, because of my travel schedule and the number of meals that I wind up eating in a restaurant, I modified this to be one "junk" meal per week. This was harder to manage and did create some slipping in my habits.

3. Cheating must be in limited quantity. I love chocolate. I cannot imagine life without it, but as I described earlier in the book, I was a sugar addict. I drank four to six Cokes every day and ate M&M's by the cup-full. Sugar had a severe impact on my immune system and I simply had to end the addiction.

   Once I stopped consuming sugar, I found that I didn't feel like I had finished my meals, particularly lunch, unless I had something sweet at the end. I felt unsatisfied and I continued to feel hungry. It was as if my body needed a sweet morsel to bookend my meal.

   For me, this was a slippery slope indeed. A sweet morsel could easily turn into an entire Butterfinger or a piece of pecan pie. Fortunately, the candy industry began individually wrapping *sweet morsels* years ago. In addition, I knew that I could have another one tomorrow after lunch and the urge to have six or seven Nestle Crunch bars was no longer so severe. Now that this is a habit, I do not think twice about having a single sweet morsel and nothing more.

Do I need to repeat a week if I don't follow the behavior changes in my PRRT Table six times that week?
If it is week 2, 3 or 4, use your judgment. If you only checked the box in the PRRT table two or three times, you should probably repeat the week. If you don't get six checks in weeks 5, 6 or 7, I suggest you repeat the week. Repetition is critical to retraining the body.

Do you think that people should reward themselves at important milestones?
The two strongest motivators for adults are fear and greed. Fear happens to be a stronger motivator than greed, but if you are not that motivated by fear of chronic illness (as I am), or if you need something more near-term and tangible to keep you motivated, then I recommend you use rewards. If this describes you, I recommend that you reward yourself at the end of each PRRT Table week where you have six check marks. Consider buying new kitchen equipment when you adopt your new eating habits or buying some new clothes to show off your figure when you reach a certain activity goal.

What do I do with the routines that were my cues for performing a certain behavior change after I complete week 7?

I suggest that you keep the cues that you know help to keep you on track. For me, routines are what keep me consistent. I would be a mess without my routines.

What should I do at times when my routines change dramatically like on vacation or on a business trip?
Don't stop your new habits. While periodic, isolated cheating is encouraged, I strongly discourage putting your habits on pause for a vacation or business trip. Habits need their own momentum and if you stop that momentum, it is hard to get it back.

So, take your habits on the road with you. You may need to make some adjustments in your routines because of the change in your schedule, but make an effort to keep the momentum of your habits going. You can do it.

What should I do if I notice that I am slipping and beginning to lose a Habit of Health?
Most importantly, don't panic and don't get discouraged. Even after you have changed your habits, you will slip up. Remember – it's a process, not an event.

The world around you, unfortunately, tends to reinforce bad habits, not good ones. And there are certain habits that you will always need to be vigilant about. For me, it is getting enough rest. My family and professional commitments tend to be greater than my waking hours, so I am often tempted to steal time from sleep.

If it has been less than 30 days since you fell off of the wagon, you simply need to recommit yourself to the habit and begin following it again. Your body will quickly re-adopt the habit as it is the stimulus it is accustomed to expect (the Habit of Health still has momentum).Typically, it takes less than a week to get back into autopilot with your Habit of Health.

If it has been more than 30 days since you fell off of the wagon, you will probably need to go back through the PRRT process again to readopt the habit. Your body and brain have probably adapted to a new habit or set of habits.

Chapter 15

True Health

He who has health has hope; and he who has hope has everything.
Arabian Proverb

"You need to get home here right away," she sobbed. "It can't wait until the weekend."

When you hear someone that you have known for decades cry for the very first time, it really gets your attention. It was the first day of 2007 and I had called to wish my Dad a Happy New Year. It wasn't a Happy New Year.

Over the last year, the complications from my Dad's cancer had landed him in the hospital seven or eight times. He had infections that wouldn't go away, catheters that collapsed, bowels that refused to work, incredible nausea that caused him to lose 60 pounds, sores all over his scalp and in his mouth and throat from the chemotherapy drugs, blood clots, hallucinations, sleepless days and nights, constant pain from the tumor in his hip and various and sundry other nagging medical issues. Incredibly, as everyone around him recalls, he never complained – not one time. Dad never wanted to make people feel bad, not even for sympathy, and he vowed never to complain.

In October of 2006, his doctor from Sloan Kettering Cancer Center had called with news that a new drug had been released and it seemed tailor made for Dad's cancer. It was specifically for metastatic colon cancer patients who had "failed chemotherapy." It was among a new class of drugs that inhibited the growth of cancer cells by targeting certain enzymes that this type of cancer needed to grow and reproduce. The clinical trial numbers were impressive and Dad switched to the new drug immediately.

Although Dad had been in the hospital a lot leading up to Christmas 2006, we were very optimistic. His tumor markers had decreased and we felt that we had gotten the miracle for which we had all been praying. The nausea had caused him to lose a great deal of weight and his bowels had stopped working without a laxative. We concluded that this was the result of his miracle drug and it was a small price to pay.

As I drove from Atlanta up to his home in Kentucky on New Year's Day, 2007, I noticed three billboards within about an hour of each other advertising cancer treatments. I noticed two billboards advertising Cyberknife radiation at a hospital north of Atlanta and one billboard for a new cancer center in Chattanooga. I must say, it startled me. As I drove along reflecting on the surprise of the mass advertising of cancer treatments, I recalled seeing similar cancer center billboards during a recent business trip to Jacksonville, Florida. It struck me as I drove along that cancer, the world's most sinister terrorist, had quietly woven its way into the fabrics of our lives.

When I arrived at my Dad's, I found him confined to his bed, lacking the strength to sit up or stand. He was so weak, he could scarcely form words, occasionally stringing three words together. I was shocked because I had spoken to him at length on Christmas Day. I knew he was having trouble, but I had no idea that his condition was deteriorating so fast.

I called his doctors in Kentucky and New York to get their opinions. Having seen this before, they both quickly concluded that this was the cancer and not the chemotherapy. His complications, they said, had become increasingly frequent and, in their opinions, after a long and valiant fight, he was succumbing to the disease. Both men sincerely expressed their love for my Dad and their admiration for his optimism and will to live, but they agreed, separately, that it was time to bring in hospice and manage "palliation," as the end of life is medically called.

I got to talk briefly with my Dad that night about the college football bowl games and showed him recent pictures of his grandchildren. He managed to give me a wink and tell me that he loved me. By morning, he had slipped into a semi-conscious state, able only to get a nod or a whisper out here and there. Hospice came in and began to focus on making the end of his life as comfortable as possible.

A few hours later, he was gone. My father died on January 3, 2007, after a 10-year battle with cancer. He was 64.

Cancer tortures and kills millions of innocent people every year. Compared to terrorism, cancer is far more effective, statistically, and far more evil in its slow, painful methods of torture and death. Cancer is indiscriminate in its killing – young, old, male, female, white, black, Latino, rich, poor, city, country, blue collar, white collar, Christian, Muslim, Hindu, heathen – and it is ruthless in its painful and debilitating destruction of the human body. Yet, for some reason, we simply accept it as a normal state of affairs.

That day, the mortician presented us with a legal form to sign acknowledging my Dad's death. It is an odd thing to do on the day of someone's death, but that is the process, I guess. On this form, among some other pretty standard information, my father's cause of death was listed as "natural causes."

It turns out that death by "natural causes" is a loosely-defined term used by coroners to describe death when the cause of death was a "naturally occurring" disease process, or is not apparent given medical history or circumstances. Thus, deaths caused by active human intervention are excluded from this definition and are described as "unnatural deaths." As of the year 2000, the most common "natural causes" of death in the U.S. are heart disease, accounting for 30% of all deaths and cancer, accounting for an additional 25% of all deaths. Other common "natural causes" are stroke, Alzheimer's disease, congenital anomalies, genetic disorders (such as cystic fibrosis), serious infections, and respiratory disorders.

Wow. What an oxymoron. Self-inflicted cancer is a natural cause of death, but deaths "caused by active human intervention" are not considered natural causes. It seems to me that the only "natural cause" of death is when the body fails as a result of senescence. Natural death is when the human body dies from age-related illness brought on by cells reaching their Hayflick limit and being unable to regenerate. Shouldn't everything else be unnatural causes? How incredibly complacent are we that we consider self-inflicted heart disease, stroke and cancer to be "natural causes" of death? If death from self-inflicted cancer at age 64 is a "natural cause," then the Civil War was a natural disaster.

There is nothing natural about cancer and chronic, degenerative disease. There is an epidemic of degenerative disease that has changed our society in absurd ways and we have become convinced that it is somehow normal and natural. Out of 100 randomly selected Americans, statistics show that 10 have diabetes, 27 have cardiovascular disease and 33 have had or will have cancer. That is *not* normal. That is *not* natural.

Truth

Truth is so powerful. With truth, there are no shades of gray – there is only truth.

Yet, it is hard to find these days. It is typically hidden under layers of spin and opinion, filtered by social correctness and rationalized by context and circumstance. It has often been hijacked and modified by special interests in order to suit their... well... special interests.

Take global warming, for example. In the1980's, environmentalists around the world began to call attention to a human-induced phenomenon with catastrophic side-effects that became known as "global warming." If left unchecked, they said, global warming would deeply change the earth, the weather and our lives. The environmentalists claimed that our species needed to make a fundamental change in the way we lived on this planet in order to avert this crisis.

The concept was frightening and it grabbed headlines. Scientists all over the world began to suggest that the increase in human activity, most notably the burning of fossil fuels and deforestation, was the cause of most of the global warming observed since the start of the industrial era in the 1950's. People everywhere began to ask the important questions like, "How can we burn less fuel or less harmful fuel?" and, "How can we stop deforestation?"

Questions like these caused great concern for some rather influential companies around the world. The answers would most certainly be bad for their profits. Relatively quickly, a systematic campaign arose to deride and ridicule the assertions of the environmentalists. New scientific studies grabbed headlines countering the conclusions of global warming. An ongoing media debate ensued with so-called environmentalists on one side and the companies that were the major fossil fuel consumers and deforesters on the other. The environmentalists were labeled as tree-hugging, liberal, fear mongers with ulterior motives to slow human progress. Scientific "evidence" was produced to calm the population and avert the profit crisis. The corporations began to win the media campaign and the environmentalists' calls for change were largely ignored by the general populace.

Nearly three decades later, the scientific evidence and support of a global warming trend is overwhelming. It appears that the whacko, alarmist tree-huggers were right from the beginning (even if they are whacko, alarmist tree-huggers). Today, in 2008, there is general agreement among scientists around the world that global warming is real and it is largely a result of the burning of fossil fuels and deforestation. No one really knows the magnitude of the damage or how reversible it is. And no one fully understands the consequences that we will face, but we now know that our species has done serious damage to our planet.

It's a funny thing about truth. With the passage of time, it always emerges and stands alone. Truth is immutable.

It turns out that we are having to deal with a heaping helping of truth right now. The 1960's and 1970's were the age of rebellion and individualism, the 1980's and 1990's were the age of excess and the early decades of the 21st century are likely to be viewed as the age of responsibility. First we liberated our rights as individuals, then we used them in the pursuit of pleasure and possessions, and now we are seeing the consequences of our excess. As a species, we are facing a looming environmental crisis, the threat of an energy crisis and the reality of a health crisis. Whether we are ready to be responsible or not, here we are. Truth has emerged and we have to make it our business.

As it relates to health, the truth is, we are sick and getting sicker. The cumulative effect of our unhealthy habits combined with the toxicity of our planet is causing many, if not most, of our chronic, degenerative health problems. Whether or not our science is mature enough to confirm it and whether or not our profit-driven corporations benefit from it is irrelevant. The truth will stand. It always does.

I just hope it doesn't have to stand and wait too long.

My friend, Lee Collier, a survivor of metastatic melanoma (skin cancer than has spread to other locations in the body, in his case the brain and lungs) was recently in his doctor's office and overheard his doctor just outside the exam room door telling a medical resident that he could not explain Lee's survival. For those of you who don't know, metastatic melanoma, statistically speaking, is a death sentence. But it isn't for Lee. Lee has lived years since his diagnosis, beating all of the odds. And his doctors just scratch their well-educated heads.

Lee, against the advice of all of his doctors, aggressively changed his habits after his diagnosis. I met Lee after a speech I gave and he wanted to know all about The Eight Habits of Healthy People. His doctors had given him a few months to live and, as you might guess, he eagerly listened to and adopted everything I told him (to be fair, much of what I told him supported what he had read elsewhere and gave him a confirming push). He also adopted a strict supplementation regimen based on his research into metastatic cancer.

On that visit to his doctor, Lee's blood work was a little unusual and he and his doctor discussed the anomalies in his liver enzymes and his white blood cell counts. Lee shared with me that his doctor, an oncologist, strongly encouraged Lee to stop his 'crazy' health habits, as that must be what was causing the abnormalities in his blood work. "Go have a burger, eat some M&M's, Lee," his doctor urged him. "Enjoy life."

Lee agreed to stop the habits for six weeks and then returned to his doctor's office for more blood work. The results of his blood work were nearly identical and the doctors had to admit that his 'crazy' habits had nothing to do with the abnormalities in his blood work. Lee immediately started his 'crazy' habits again.

What struck me about this story was the incredible blindness of this doctor. Literally, within the same breath, he confides in his resident that he cannot explain why Lee is still alive, and then tells Lee to stop those darned 'crazy' behaviors that make him different from the other cancer patients…who died. What keeps a well-educated person, a trained scientist no less, from making the connection between statistical anomaly and unique behavior? How can this person be so blind to cause and effect as to suggest that Lee stop the thing that is keeping him alive while the vast majority of the people stricken with his condition die?

The answer is science and profit. I know it sounds like a conspiracy theory, but just think about it. Consider the possibility that the profit motive of corporate interests misuse science as a tool to suppress truth. Think it can't happen? Reread the story on global warming above.

I am not suggesting that Lee's doctor – or any doctor or group of doctors or company or group of companies or board of directors or group of shareholders – is executing a well-orchestrated plan to suppress the truth about our health using science. What I am suggesting is that profit growth is a singular corporate goal that overpowers all other goals including human interest and that science, like statistics, is a tool that is used for its gain and protection.

On September 11, 2001, terrorists attacked the World Trade Center. The United States government and governments around the world have spent billions of your dollars chasing down those responsible for the 2,996 deaths that resulted from those attacks. In 2007, melanoma killed 8,110 people. If healthcare is about caring for our health, why isn't there a team of scientists studying Lee? Shouldn't someone from the Centers for Disease Control headquarters drive to see Lee at his doctor's office at Emory University Hospital and ask a few questions… 2.4 miles away?

Facts are facts. Lee is beating overwhelming odds and Lee follows a series of health habits that most people with his diagnosis do not. The truth is standing and waiting for us to acknowledge it. How long does it have to wait?

Health, Really
In 2006, *USA Today* reported that one in three Americans said that their greatest fear in old age is experiencing health problems. The second most quoted concern about old age was not having enough money and a distant third concern was dying. Imagine that – Americans are more concerned about poor health in old age than they are about actually dying.

Simply stated, *health* is the absence of sickness. To say that someone has his health is to say that he is free from sickness. *Healthcare* is any activity that promotes or maintains the state of health. Said another way, *healthcare* is a proactive activity to preserve the state of being free from sickness. The stuff in this book (and in other resources like it), is advice on *healthcare*.

Unfortunately, the medical industry got to pick its name first, and it settled on the term "healthcare." In reality, though, the stuff that most people think of when they think of *healthcare* – the doctors, hospitals and drugs – is really *sick care*. Legendary economist Paul Zane Pilzer has written, "What we call the 'healthcare' business is really the sickness business. The $1.4 trillion we spend on medical care is concerned with treating the symptoms of sickness. It has very little to do with being stronger or healthier."

In contrast to the definition of healthcare above, sick care is a reactive activity to resolve or mitigate the state of sickness. And although most in the sick care business would label the advice in this book as *alternative medicine* or *wellness*, there is nothing *alternative* about the daily habits that one follows to maintain his health. In fact, I would argue that the doctors, hospitals and drugs are *alternatives* to the daily habits that one follows to maintain his health. As for the label "*wellness*," I don't really know what that means, but it always makes me think of long beards, flowing robes, crystals and incense. At best, it sounds more like a destination than an activity and, therefore, could not encompass the daily habits that one follows to maintain his health.

To be clear, this book is not a recommendation for anyone to abandon their doctor's care or ignore their advice. It is an encouragement for you to become the CEO of your health and be responsible and accountable for it. Think of and treat your doctors as advisors in your health. You should be in charge of the decisions regarding your health, but like any good CEO, you consult with your advisors, the specialists, before making your decision. I feel sure that none of them will tell you that adopting healthy habits is a bad idea.

To keep your health, you must take control of it and be responsible for it. That means not simply giving your care over to some doctor that you have spent a total of six to ten hours with in your whole life. Do you put your financial future entirely into your banker's hands? Do you put your professional future entirely into your boss's hands? Probably not. So why would you put your health and your future entirely into the hands of a doctor whom you barely know?

Your doctor is not going to obsess over the long-term side effects of a drug he prescribes for you to take for the rest of your life. Your personal trainer is not going to obsess over the quality of the water you drink or the synthetic chemicals in your food. Your pharmacist is not going to obsess over length and quality of your sleep or the amount of stress in your life. You have to.

Clearly the sick care business – the doctors, hospitals, pharmacies and drug companies – are effective at caring for sickness. So, when you are sick or have experienced trauma, go see the experts. Sick care is what they do – and they do a very good job at it.

However, the sick care business does not have a big role in health care (that is, in maintaining your health). You play the biggest role in maintaining your state of health. (The role that the sick care business can play in helping you maintain your health is primarily a measurement role because of its very advanced diagnostic capabilities.)

Your health is your business. It is *your* business. You have to be responsible for your choices. No one else will. Your health is your responsibility and you should not put it in the hands of someone else; not a doctor, not a pharmacist, not a hospital, not a drug company, not a vitamin company, not a personal trainer, not an herbalist, not a chiropractor, not anyone. No one is going to look out for your health as vigilantly as you will (or should).

Health is a Choice
We are beginning to learn that our bodies are not as hardy and resilient as we would like to believe. Humans, like their planet, live in delicate harmony that can easily be disrupted. In the same way that our planet's balance has been disturbed by the continuous burning of its fossil fuels and deforestation, our bodies' balance has been disturbed by a continuous barrage of foreign chemicals and unhealthy living.

Like the damage to our planet, no one really knows the magnitude or reversibility of the damage that each of us has done to our body, but one thing appears certain. The cumulative impact of the deterioration results in an array of diseases that is overwhelming mankind.

As a young man, I followed unhealthy habits that resulted in a depressed immune system. I ate too much sugar, ate a diet high in processed food and animal fat, and I rarely drank water. As a typical American boy growing up in the 1970's and 1980's, I frequently came into contact with toxic chemicals and I did not follow habits that helped me to rid my body of those toxins. With a weakened immune system unable to fight off the molecular malfunctions resulting from the increasing toxic load in my body, I developed cancer. Looking back, it shouldn't have been a surprise. I had put together the perfect recipe for sickness – The Cumulative Effect.

Fortunately, the sick care industry had a remedy for my sickness and my tumors were eradicated. However, no one taught me how to address the cause of my sickness and I continued my unhealthy habits even after my cancer went into remission. Having a deadly disease has a way of causing you to evaluate a lot of things, especially your health. And as I assessed my health, I became convinced that I was destined to die from disease unless I could find a way to prevent it from recurring.

Over the next twenty years, as I studied human health in an effort to find a way to avoid more disease, I discovered that the tools for living a healthy life were not in some pharmacy, health food store or hospital. The tools for living a healthy life are *inside* of us. I discovered that the "doctor" that lives within each of us is more knowledgeable than any scientific or technological advance that our minds have ever conceived of, and I found that the habits that we choose to follow every day not only make up the fiber of who we are, but they determine the very health of our bodies.

I discovered that there are no magic potions that create health and there are no silver bullets that destroy it. Very simply, human health is determined by our habits. Because our routine, habitual actions account for 80% - 90% of the actions that affect our health, focusing on adopting and following healthier habits has a far greater impact on health than anything else that we can do. More specifically, I discovered that human health in the modern context depends upon a set of habits that consistently:
1. Reduce your exposure to harmful toxins
2. Rid your body of the toxins it does encounter
3. Fortify your immune system
4. Maintain the health of your body's life-supporting systems

The eight habits outlined in this book do all four of these very important things for you. Done in combination, these habits will provide a lifetime of protection against the epidemic of degenerative disease.

And although they may feel automatic, your habits are a choice. No matter how long you have followed your current routine, you can change your habits. And if you can form new habits – habits of health – you can change your health and your life.

Choosing to be healthy is no longer an abstract concept. If your habits determine your health and your habits are a choice, it follows then that health is a choice. This book gives you very specific tools to help you adopt a new set of habits that will forever change your health. You now have the information you need to operate the human machine in the modern environment and the tools to apply it.

It is time to choose to be healthy.

Choose
I'm a worrier, but a lot has changed about my worries. I went from being convinced that I was going to die of cancer and living a life in fear of every spot, lump and cough to being concerned that I was not saving enough for retirement because I became sure that I would live into my 90's. My views of the world and of my body have completely changed. I think of food, rest, water and exercise as medicine and my immune system as the doctor most qualified to treat my ailments. My new plan is to be around to see all of my children reach retirement and be a source of inspiration and support when they hit the tough patches along the way.

I challenge you to take control of your health and begin to live your life with the satisfaction and confidence that only true health can bring you. I dare you to live your life with the worries that you will run out of retirement and wear out your body from use. I invite you to commit yourself to seeing your children retire and your grandchildren's children take their first steps.

If I could reach out right now, through the pages of this book, I'd grasp your shoulders with my two hands and say, "Use your judgment. Use your common sense. Your health is the most precious gift that God has given you. The choice is yours to make and you must make that choice right now and every day from now on."

Seize this moment in time. Make the decision to be *impatient* instead of *a patient.*

Sources

Introduction
Pritikin, Robert. Live Long, Live Well

Chapter 1: The Epidemic Secret
US Department of Health
The American Heart Association
The National Center for Health Statistics
The National Institutes for Health
The Centers for Disease Control & Prevention
The American Stroke Association
Pritikin, Robert. Live Long, Live Well
Wired May, 2004
Rubin, Jordan. The Maker's Diet
www.wikipedia.com
http://www.wwu.edu/depts/healthyliving/PE511info/arthritis/arthritis
_statistics.htm
Oz, Mehmet and Michael F. Roizen. YOU: The Owner's Manual

Chapter 2: How Science and Profit Abducted Health
Grace, Kelly. "The New View of Health." Experience Life Magazine
Colbert, Don. Walking In Divine Health
www.wikipedia.com
Bernstein, Elizabeth. "Holy Mackerel! Fish Is Good." Wall Street
Journal October 18, 2006
McCain, John. Character is Destiny
Lueck, Sarah. "Health-Care Spending Growth Slows." Wall Street Journal
January 10, 2006
"The World in 2006, The World In Figures." The Economist
"Medicare Makes Room For Medicine Chest." Wall Street Journal
November 26th, 2006
"Health, United States 2004." U.S. Government Report
Matthews, Anna Wilde. "At Medical Journals, Writers Paid By Industry
Play Big Role." Wall Street Journal December 13, 2006
Armstrong, David. "Cleveland Clinic Had Ties To Maker of Faulted
Device" Wall Street Journal December 16, 2005
Martinez, Barbara "Merck Expects to Resume Earnings Growth in
2007." Wall Street Journal December 16, 2005

Chapter 3: The Cumulative Effect
International numbers provided by the Census Bureau
Domestic numbers from the National Center for Health Statistics
http://en.wikipedia.org/wiki/Pima
Price, Weston. "Nutrition and Physical Degeneration." Price-Pottenger
Foundation 1939, 1997
Colbert, Don Toxic Relief

Chapter 4: Health 102
Weil, Andrew. Spontaneous Healing videocassette
Bricklin, Mark. The Practical Encyclopedia of Natural Healing 983
Soukup, Elise. "Periscope" Newsweek January 2, 2006

Chapter 5: Live on Nature's Harvest
The American Lung Association
The Centers for Disease Control & Prevention
The National Center for Health Statistics
U.S. Department of Health & Human Services, Public Health Service.
The Surgeon General's Report on Nutrition and Health 1988
Pollan, Michael. The Omnivore's Dilemma: A Natural History of Four
Meals
http://www.mypyramid.gov/pyramid/grains_tips.html
www.mypyramid.gov/pyramid/vegetables_tips.html
http://www.mypyramid.gov/pyramid/fruits_tips.html
http://www.mypyramid.gov/pyramid/meat_tips.html
http://us.cnn.com/HEALTH/library/HQ/00599.html
www.cancer.org
Weil, Andrew. Eating For Optimum Health videocassette
Rubin, Jordan. The Maker's Diet
S. Lindberg and B. Lundh. "Apparent Absence of Stroke and Ischaemic
Heart Disease in a Traditional Melanesian Island: A Clinical Study of
Kitava"
http://beans4health.org
Peck, Peggy. "Five Servings of Fruits and Vegetables Dip Stroke Risk"
www.cnn.com
Colbert, Don Toxic Relief
Prevention Plus Fall/ Winter 2005
http://www.mypyramid.gov/pyramid/fruits_why.html
Rosenbloom, Chris. "A More Colorful Diet is a Step In The Right
Direction." Atlanta Journal and Constitution January 5, 2006
Weil, Andrew. Eight Weeks to Optimum Health

http://www.mypyramid.gov/pyramid/grains.html
Colbert, Don. Walking In Divine Health
http://www.mypyramid.gov/pyramid/meat_why.html
American Journal of Clinical Nutrition
Annals of Internal Medicine October, 1998
Annals of Internal Medicine March, 2003
The New England Journal of Medicine July, 2004

Chapter 6: Drink From The Fountain of Health:
United States Environmental Protection Agency "Total Maximum Daily
Load Evaluation for Seven Segments of the Chattahoochee River in the
Chattahoochee River Basin (PCBs in Fish Tissue)." 1997
www.aquasana.com
Carlton, Jim. "Cities Spend Millions on Land to Protect Water." Wall
Street Journal January 4, 2006
http://www.internethealthlibrary.com/Environmental-Health/Chlorine-
and-cancer.htm
http://www.nrdc.org/health/kids/ocar/chap7.asp
http://www.internethealthlibrary.com/Environmental-Health/Chlorine-
and-cancer.htm
http://www.nrdc.org/health/kids/ocar/chap7.asp
http://www.internethealthlibrary.com/Environmental-Health/Chlorine-
and-cancer.htm

Chapter 7: Be In-Dependent
The American Cancer Society. "Facts & Figures 2003." 2003
Tashkin, Donald. Presentation to the American Thoracic Society
Conference, May 23 2006
www.cancer.org
Colbert, Don. What You Don't Know May Be Killing You
"Tipple Play." Sky Magazine August, 2005
"Drinking Joins Smoking as Cancer Risk." www.cnn.com January 30,
2006
Archives of Internal Medicine 1H 2006

Chapter 8: Use Your Body
The Centers for Disease Control & Prevention
The American Heart Association
The American Cancer Society
Parker-Pope, Tara. "Why Your New Year's Resolution to Get Healthier
May Be Pretty Easy to Keep." Wall Street Journal

Pritikin, Robert. Live Long, Live Well
Colbert, Don. What You Don't Know May Be Killing You
The Journal of Gerontology: Medical Sciences November, 2006

Chapter 9: Carry the Right Weight
The National Institutes of Health
The Centers for Disease Control and Prevention
The National Center for Health Statistics
The American Cancer Society
The American Lung Association
Washington Business Group on Health
Weight Control Information Network
Crawford, Kristen. "The Big Opportunity." Business 2.0 June, 2006
Obesity Research Journal
Colbert, Don. Toxic Relief
Pollan, Michael. The Omnivore's Dilemma: A Natural History of Four Meals
Pritikin, Robert. Live Long, Live Well
Duncan, Emma. "The World In 2006." The Economist
Annals of Internal Medicine January 3, 2006
Oz, Mehmet and Michael F. Roizen. YOU: The Owner's Manual
Dooren, Jennifer Corbett., "Carbs May Not Weigh You Down." Wall Street Journal January 4, 2006

Chapter 10: Live an Organic Life
The Harvard School of Public Health
Biotechnology Industry Organization
The United States Department of Agriculture, Economic Research Service
Pollan, Michael. The Omnivore's Dilemma: A Natural History of Four Meals
Colbert, Don. Toxic Relief
Annals of Neurology July, 2006
Wired May, 2004
Colbert, Don. Walking In Divine Health
Gray, Steven. "Organic Food Goes Mass Market." Wall Street Journal May 4, 2006
Owen, James. "Farming Claims Almost Half Earth's Land, New Maps Show." National Geographic News December 9, 2005
Bounds, Gwendolyn and Ilan Brat. "Turf Wars" Wall Street Journal April 15, 2006

http://www.healthgoods.com/Education/Healthy_Home_Information/
Home_Health_Hazards/hazardous_products.htm
http://www.ecomall.com/greenshopping/epasafe22.htm
Colbert, Don. What You Don't Know May Be Killing You
Rubin, Jordan. The Maker's Diet

Chapter 11: Detox Your Body
Rubin, Jordan. The Maker's Diet
Colbert, Don. Toxic Relief
http://www.holisticmed.com/detox/dtx-intro.txt
Colbert, Don. What You Don't Know May Be Killing You
www.aquasaua.com
http://www.chetday.com/spencedetox.html
http://www.holisticmed.com/detox/detox.html
Ford, Alyssa. "Start Seeing Toxins" Experience Life May, 2007
Oz, Mehmet and Michael F. Roizen. YOU: The Owner's Manual
http://www.juicefasting.org/juicefasting.htm
http://www.healingdaily.com/juicing-for-health/fasting.htm

Chapter 12: Rest & Relax
Oz, Mehmet and Michael F. Roizen. YOU: The Owner's Manual
http://www.bettersleep.org
Irwin, M., McClintick, J., Costlow, C., Fortner, M., White, J., Gum, J. C.
"Partial night sleep deprivation reduces natural killer and cellular immune
responses in humans." Departments of Psychiatry, University of
California, and San Diego Veterans Affairs Medical Center
www.wikipedia.com
http://www.stress.org

Chapter 13: Make a Plan
http://www.zenhabits.net

Diagnosed with cancer at the age of 18, Matt McConnell faced down death at an early age. After undergoing surgery and several rounds of chemotherapy, the disease went into remission. However, he remained in poor health throughout his young adult life. Convinced that he would again have to face the disease, McConnell made the decision to take control of his health and threw himself into the study of preventative medicine.

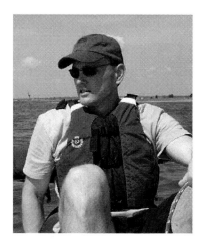

For over twenty years, Matt studied and experimented with a broad variety of health practices in order to improve his body's ability to fight sickness. Through extensive trial and error, he identified eight relatively simple habits that dramatically improved his health, allowing him to live without a symptom of illness of any kind.

Astonished by his complete health transformation, McConnell became convinced that sickness and, ultimately, degenerative disease could be prevented through the adoption of these eight fairly simple changes in lifestyle. Confident that his results could be duplicated by people around the world, Matt refined the routines that had transformed his own health and married them with an innovative method for habit adoption that he helped to develop in his professional life. In *Get Well Soon: The Eight Habits of Healthy People*, McConnell is able to combine his passion and knowledge for health with his expertise in human behavior.

Matt is the founder, Chairman and Chief Executive Officer of Knowlagent, Inc, a leading provider of software for developing human capital. He is married, has three children and lives outside of Atlanta, Georgia.

Notes